PUBLIC HEALTH AND BEYOND IN LATIN AMERICA AND THE CARIBBEAN

Public Health and Beyond in Latin America and the Caribbean: Reflections from the Field explores the diverse and complex public health landscape, from global to regional to local, by considering historical and socio-cultural factors to contextualize the ongoing public health crisis.

Drawing on four decades of field experience, research, and teaching, Sherri L. Porcelain uses case studies to offer a realistic view of the public heath struggle in Latin America and the Caribbean. Using specific countries as regional examples, the book shows how population health has been inextricably linked to political, economic, social, cultural, ethical, ecological, environmental, and technological factors. Chapters in this book will examine the history of public health issues associated with international development, globalization and the international political economy, disasters, diplomacy, and security studies coupled with the changing role of key actors driving the global and regional agendas. The final chapter examines the impact of the COVID-19 pandemic and what it means for the future of public health.

This book is recommended for undergraduate students interested in the history of Latin America and the Caribbean as well as others concerned with global and regional population health challenges.

Sherri L. Porcelain is a Lecturer in the Department of International Studies at the University of Miami where she teaches global public health in world affairs with a focus on Latin America and the Caribbean for the Interdisciplinary International Studies Program. She has also been a voluntary faculty member in the Department of Public Health Sciences at the university since 1988.

Latin American Tópicos
Edited by Michael LaRosa, Rhodes College

For more information about this series, please visit: www.routledge.com/
Latin-American-Tpicos/book-series/LAT

PUBLIC HEALTH AND BEYOND IN LATIN AMERICA AND THE CARIBBEAN

Reflections from the Field

Sherri L. Porcelain

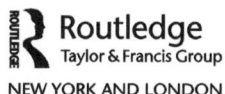

Routledge
Taylor & Francis Group

NEW YORK AND LONDON

First published 2022
by Routledge
605 Third Avenue, New York, NY 10158

and by Routledge
2 Park Square, Milton Park, Abingdon, Oxon, OX14 4RN

Routledge is an imprint of the Taylor & Francis Group, an informa business

Library of Congress Cataloging-in-Publication Data
Names: Porcelain, Sherri L., author.
Title: Public health and beyond in Latin America and the Caribbean :
reflections from the field / Sherri L. Porcelain.
Description: First edition. | New York, NY : Routledge, 2022. |
Series: Latin american tópicos | Includes bibliographical references
and index.
Identifiers: LCCN 2021014801 (print) | LCCN 2021014802 (ebook) |
ISBN 9780367440756 (paperback) | ISBN 9780367440763 (hardback) |
ISBN 9781003007401 (ebook)
Subjects: LCSH: Medical care—Latin America. | Medical
care—Caribbean.
Classification: LCC RA450.5 .P68 2022 (print) |
LCC RA450.5 (ebook) | DDC 362.1098—dc23
LC record available at https://lccn.loc.gov/2021014801
LC ebook record available at https://lccn.loc.gov/2021014802

ISBN: 978-0-367-44076-3 (hbk)
ISBN: 978-0-367-44075-6 (pbk)
ISBN: 978-1-003-00740-1 (ebk)

DOI: 10.4324/9781003007401

Typeset in Bembo
by codeMantra

CONTENTS

ACKNOWLEDGMENTS

My heartfelt thank you to Michael LaRosa, series editor for Tópicos, first for his encouragement to write this book, and second for his unwavering commitment to read and offer suggestions through the drafts of this book. Also, great appreciation to assistant editor, Emily Irvine, who was always there with gentle reminders and answers to my questions, along with the precision offered by senior editor, Kimberley Smith and the Production Manager Sashivadana and the Codemantra team. A very special thank you to Valerie Gramling, University of Miami professor in the English Department for her valuable assistance, and to Lisa Baker, head librarian for international studies, for helping me to find the hard to locate materials. I would be remiss if I did not recognize Omar Gilzean, supervisor for technical support, for saving me from a meltdown while reconciling my files after a distressing computer crash in the midst of a pandemic and while writing this manuscript.

The unique contributions to this book were made possible by the talented artist, Karina Rojas, whom I have worked with on numerous post disaster public health projects and former student Sofia Mohammad for her creative maps, offering their unique perspectives. I also acknowledge the contributions of Ali Habashi, a professor and documentary filmmaker in the School of Communication, for teaching me to become more discerning about selecting images to effectively communicate messages. It is his skillful eye that captured the image on the cover of this book.

My gratitude to Juana Herrera for her decades of friendship and trust in working together.

This book implies that it is the work of a single author, while the truth is that the contributions are too numerous to recount. Over the many decades, I've learned to appreciate that any project, academic or not, is shaped by our formal or more casual interactions. For this, I acknowledge the many names faded in my memory while their faces and indomitable spirits have guided me in writing this book.

Last but not least is the recognition that none of my travels, expeditions, and sometimes last minute field work would have been possible without the support of my husband, Dan Forman, for also "holding down the fort" – of course, with much support when our children were young. It takes a village.

PREFACE

This book is the outcome of more than four decades of learning, researching, and engaging in field experiences related to public health, disasters, or community development projects across different populations in Latin America and the Caribbean. I was reluctant to write, analyze, and share my "personal" experiences as case studies and reflections from the field, since I felt this could be interpreted as self-serving and potentially disrespectful to the many resilient people who taught me about the human face of population health, safety, and security. I was encouraged by the Tópicos series editor, Michael LaRosa, that such hands-on experiences coupled with the historical and empirical evidence would be a worthy contribution to undergraduate students studying the history of Latin America and the Caribbean as well others concerned with global and regional population health challenges. History has shown us that public health matters, and we must recognize that better outcomes are unmistakable when the attention reaches beyond the narrow focus of "health" in public health.

Writing about the complexities of public health was already a daunting task. Then the pandemic arrived. COVID-19, lamentably, underscores why this global to regional to national public health challenge is necessarily interconnected to many academic disciplines, perspectives, and underlying issues that impact livelihoods and the health of peoples. This book explores the idealization of global public health with an earnest effort to elucidate how the internal and external factors will influence or become influenced by social, economic, and political development, globalization, disasters and climate crisis, diplomacy, and security. It concludes by showing how each of these themes, presented as separate chapters, help to shape the public health conundrum. While each topic is fundamental to analyzing the COVID-19 pandemic, history reminds us that it is only when they are pieced together that a complete picture is created. It is my intent to exemplify this broader image of (global) public health with a focus on Latin America and the Caribbean. Perhaps, to some, this is a caricature. This is for you to question.

Sherri L. Porcelain
March 15, 2021

INTRODUCTION

A review of some Latin America and the Caribbean regional public health challenges throughout history, for example, from the deadly diseases of yellow fever, malaria, and cholera, thwarting the French from successfully building the Panama Canal in the late 19th century, to the more contemporary regional vector-borne and water-borne diseases in the Americas, cannot be studied in isolation of the rightly and relevant internal and external influences. This book is not intended to be a comprehensive review of the history of public health in Latin America and the Caribbean. For this I will refer readers to the excellent work of Marcos Cueto and Steven Palmer's 2014 text, *Medicine and Public Health in Latin America: A History*.[1]. Chapter 1 introduces the concept of public health and social and environmental determinants in Latin America and the Caribbean. Chapter 2 examines the intersection of social and economic development and how the underlying determinants of health are applied in the Americas. Chapter 3 explores the positive and detrimental effects of globalization, trade, and foreign direct investment with both the direct and indirect influences on population health, adding the commercial determinants of health to the expanded analysis. Chapter 4 discusses the intersection of disasters, climate crisis, and public health with increasing frequency and intensities of emergency events causing havoc across Latin America and the Caribbean countries and territories. Chapter 5 reframes the discussion on diplomacy and population health with a more seamless transition to regional cooperation and trust of old and new international actors. Chapter 6 explores why public health threats have become securitized overtime to become situated within the wider discussion of regional and global affairs. Chapter 7, conclusion, will briefly examine the complexities of the COVID-19 pandemic in the Americas, using each chapter

DOI: 10.4324/9781003007401-1

to show the broader relationship of economic and social development, globalization and trade, disasters, diplomacy, and security to public health within and across countries in the region.

I realize some will criticize my analysis as very broad, label it tainted by selective experiences, and recognize that it does not fully assess the region. It would be presumptuous to assume I know all the issues, populations, strategies, and policies undertaken to improve population welfare in such a diversified region. What 42 years of experiences in a few countries in the region uncovered was the realization that the more I experienced, the more I learned, or read, the less I truthfully understood. I did learn that a wider approach to public health is built upon listening more to the voices of people. I invite the reader to justly question the trajectory of public health and its wider relationships to the history of Latin America and the Caribbean and international affairs as conceptualized in this book.

I emphasize two important points for the reader. First, I include my reflections from the field, recognizing that these are my personal experiences that might reveal a bias in selecting one case study, example, or anecdote over another. Such preferences may also be related to the specific topic, time in history, place, and the people and organizations in which I interacted that have influenced the way I interpret and present my experiences throughout the book. Second, I may not have included important Latin America and Caribbean scholars, scientists, and practitioners who have added significantly to the diverse subject areas. It is not my intent to minimize their noteworthy contributions. Suitably, my intent is to present an outsider's perspective considering the history, evidence, and competing viewpoints within and across Latin America and the Caribbean.

Latin America and the Caribbean

Latin America and the Caribbean is different within and across countries. South America with 14 countries, Central America with 7 countries, and Mexico as part of the North American region. The Caribbean has 13 countries of which Cuba, Dominican Republic and Haiti (Hispaniola) speak Spanish and Creole, respectively. Not to forget Puerto Rico in the Caribbean which is a U.S. territory. Population density in 2019 spans from the smallest in the Caribbean ranging from 5,300 people in Montserrat to more than 11 million in Cuba, with Brazil as the most densely populated country in Latin America with 211.1 million followed by Mexico with 127.6 million.[2] The main languages spoken in Latin America are Spanish, Portuguese, and more than 500 Indigenous languages, with English, Dutch, French, and Haitian Creole in the Caribbean. Many Indigenous languages remain important to this region's common history of European invasions and annexation of lands that began in the late 15th century and continued through the 18th century. Latin America and the Caribbean is characterized by the multicultural, multiracial, and multiethnic countries; yet regional approaches are useful in identifying some prevailing themes in the broader discussion of population well-being.

To exemplify, health care delivery systems in Latin America and the Caribbean, beyond the Western or allopathic systems, reflect upon the important aspects of history, culture, religion, and societal/traditional practices that run parallel, are tolerant, or fully integrated into such systems. It is meaningful to know how people seek advice or use treatments outside the formal health sector, especially in the prevention and promotion of a holistic approach to mental, social, and physical well-being. Traditional healers like curandero/a practice *curanderismo* have played an important part in the Latin American culture, while ritual cleansing, *despojó*, used by *Santeria* or other religious or cultural practices in the Caribbean is considered as part of the prevention and healing processes.

Public health plays an important role in the well-being, safety, and security of a society. Many scholars, across the different fields of study, provide insightful research to support how a healthier population produces a more economically productive and politically stable society. However, in order to translate this information into effective public policies we need to rethink the way public health is perceived. This requires more attention to the wider relationship of social and environmental determinants of health as well as the commercial determinants where structural barriers have had both direct and indirect impact on the health, safety, and security of peoples. Latin America and the Caribbean has a long history of studying and understanding such problems, while the responses continue to be unequal throughout the region.

The aim of each chapter is to expand the discussion beyond a focus of "health" in population-based health issues. I hope to show why a more holistic approach – using transdisciplinary methods – is instructive. This offers the intellectual space for the greater participation of many disciplines and methodologies in response to the real-world population health, safety, and security matters.

Medical and allied health fields must not subjugate the importance of other sectors, disciplines, and perspectives, which may be rushed to consider as an afterthought. This happens way too often. Not one perspective, not one determinant, not a single discipline can tackle population health and welfare alone, albeit the medical and public health stakeholders play critical roles. I've seen communities faced with health-related problems requiring better leadership and the stewardship for continuity, and rarely did the health sector have the capabilities to tackle these alone.

I have collaborated with indigenous populations in Latin America and understood that reliable infrastructure is not always sustainable. Potable water systems may be built, while they are often breached due to the design, lack of low-cost spare parts, and bad weather which result in outbreaks of diarrheal disease as children drink untreated water and families struggle to find water for cooking and bathing. All these problems may be due to lack of one PVC piping, a filter, or political entanglements. These economic, political, and technological factors are important to the public health conundrum. The official data show potable water is available, while it is not consistently and reliably accessible. Safe water is necessary for life, important to human development, a social determinant of health, and yet not a reality for all. The concern is motivating leaders to "talk the talk and walk the walk," and not look at the temporary simple solutions that often have limited sustainable impact. The PVC pipe water system to a remote village in Panama is not the sole responsibility of the Ministry of Health. It includes other ministries, multilateral financial institutions, which funded the project, the private sector, and their partnerships with community people and leaders where all stakeholders have a voice in responding to the issues. This is not an easy task; yet there are solutions with the political will to prioritize such time and investments. Nevertheless, it is evident that the availability and accessibility to mobile phones, and yes, smart phones, have reached faster and further into regions of the world than the arrival of safe water, sanitation, and housing. In the 1980s, I asked the same questions about how liters of Coca-Cola bottles reached the most remote areas in Colombia and thought about the ingenuity of the marketing and distribution strategies of multinational corporations in a globalizing world.

The need to provide potable water, sanitation, housing, and nutrition is not the exclusive responsibility of the health sector; yet these are the foundations of a more resilient public health system. The United States learned important lessons in the late 1800s and early 1900s about the significance of investing in public health improvements. These are lessons that seem to be forgotten today as cities around the United States confront the tragic neglect of their public health infrastructure. In response to the pestilence and filth that plagued cities in the early 20th century, England, Wales, and the United States created the political will to invest in the essential infrastructure that would provide safer water, sanitation, housing, roads, and nutrition. These investments became the fundamental building blocks to many public health successes. Nevertheless, in the post-WWII era, the United States focused on a hurried mixed bag of strategies to help its neighbors to the South, rather than place the attention toward constructing a sustainable public health infrastructure as a priority. In the postwar era, through the 1970s, the focus of attention was on vaccines and antibiotics as the best response to old and new disease threats, while the lack of investment in clean water, disposal of human waste and refuse, and appropriate protective housing with safe roads was not implemented equally throughout Latin America and the Caribbean.

Then the 1980s arrived with a call for lifestyle changes and a shift away from the focus on infectious diseases toward chronic disease prevention. Nevertheless, the communicable disease burden continues to disproportionately impact numerous communities in Latin America and the Caribbean, creating a double burden of disease profile. Through these decades of progress no one will argue that great developments in urban and rural infrastructure were made in Latin America and the Caribbean, albeit unequally, though health disparities continued to present challenges. The failure to construct a sound public health foundation remains a prevailing theme and a critical lesson for sustainable health and development. Such topics are further analyzed in Chapters 1 and 2, where we see Latin America and the Caribbean continue to experience demographic, epidemiologic, nutrition, and health transitions, with rising cases of noncommunicable diseases such as cancers, heart disease, stroke, and diabetes as populations continue to age. Therefore, the profile of disease patterns shifted away from communicable to increased noncommunicable diseases throughout the region.[3] In 1989, Frenk et al. recognized that such health transitions in the middle-income countries presented new challenges for the health care systems in Latin America.[4] While medical, social and behavioral, and ecological approaches help us to explore such public health challenges, it is also the international political economy that provokes important questions about power, distribution, and the allocation of resources and social justice in public health. This is where Chapter 3 which deals with globalization explores the positive and negative impacts on population health that transborder exchanges of goods, services, diseases, ideas, knowledge, mores, and values, all of which takes place through trade, travel, tourism, and the wider communication interactions.

Health care delivery systems confront rapidly rising rates of morbidity and mortality related to heart disease, high blood pressure, diabetes, cancer, and obesity, which are competing with other public health prevention resources needed for infectious diseases, mental health, violence, and traffic-related issues. Heart disease is the number one killer followed by cancer. Diabetes has become a great public health challenge throughout the region, with increasing numbers of people overweight and obese. In 2015, it was estimated that more than 41 million people over 20 years of age were diagnosed with Type II diabetes, presenting great financial implications for the society.[5] Diabetes also contributes to cardiovascular diseases that cause heart attacks and strokes. According to the Food and Agricultural Organization of the United Nations (2019) report, 24% of the population in Latin America and the Caribbean are obese, reaching a total of 105 million people with rates tripling in both children and adolescents between 1990 and 2016.[6] The most significant rise in obesity is taking place in the Caribbean. The concern is that while obesity is rising throughout Latin America and the Caribbean, so is hunger with higher rates of undernutrition reported in the region than the global average.[7]

We need to look beyond the behaviors of peoples and explore how such structural, environmental, and commercial determinants of health are important to understanding this public health puzzle. The role and responsibility of transnational tobacco, food and beverage, and big pharmaceutical industries will be discussed, including an assessment of the commercial determinants of health and corporate social responsibility. For example, the increasing availability of highly processed foods, cheap oils, and high-sugar, obesogenic foods contributes to the nutritional transition and the soaring rates of obesity and undernutrition in the Americas. The role of trade liberalization, foreign direct investment, and promotion of a market economy are all important to the changing food and drink consumption. Brazil and Mexico are two countries in the region making strides with programs and integrated policies and tax regulations to reduce health risks, while Guatemala is seeking resources to combat malnutrition. The paradox of obesity and malnutrition throughout the Americas underscores such inequalities and health disparities within countries and across the region.

Kaleidoscopic Approach

I suggest the reader to consider a kaleidoscopic approach. Anyone who has used a kaleidoscope knows that no matter who looks through the lens, an array of images, bouncing off of the mirror reflections, will produce the varying shades of colors, shapes, sizes, and movements. Think of these images as different key actors from governmental, multilateral organizations, multilateral financial institutions, business sector, nongovernmental, religious organizations, to civil society offering their different perspectives about the complex health and health-related problems of populations. We all become better informed through collecting the different viewpoints.

I propose that the kaleidoscope is as important as the microscope is to public health. Scientists assert the necessity of a microscope, which I do not refute. However, the study and practice of public health extends beyond one lens, tool, or discipline, and need a mindful participation beyond identifying a microbe. Rethinking the image of public health provides greater insight into the organization of this book.

I first applied the term kaleidoscopic perspective shortly after Hurricane Andrew struck South Florida on August 24, 1992 around 5 am and devastated many poor farmworker residents, mostly from Mexico, Guatemala, and small states of the Caribbean residing just south of Miami in and around the city of Homestead. In response to the extensive destruction, key stakeholders presented different strategies to promote and secure the well-being of the displaced population. The critical issues of displacement and housing, safe hygiene, environmental exposures, language and cultural barriers, education, employment, along with economic and political rationales were just some of the key concerns. These are the social and environmental determinants of health that will be discussed throughout the book. Every agency and every person had a different point of view; yet, few suggestions were based upon scientific evidence or other disaster responses to support their actions. So, I used my camera and cut out images that I captured while assessing the situation to present a collage superimposed through the lens of a kaleidoscope. The way one sees the different images, shapes, sizes, and colors was portrayed in my presentation. The photos I presented were seen through the lens I used and interpreted differently by others. I, respectfully, asked the populations impacted how they felt and what they needed. I thought that we could use the official data collected and supplement with the information and collage created to recognize interpretations that could inform smart decision making? I realized that it would have been better to give displaced people disposable cameras- since smart phones were not yet available- to take pictures and capture their perspectives beyond the words they shared. I did this later on and learned so much more. We continue to confront emergency response challenges with displaced populations, and, hopefully, we have better answers than we did 29 years ago.

Chapter 4 will further explore disasters and the climate crisis in Latin America and the Caribbean that ranks the second most at-risk region in the world to disasters. Such events include floods, hurricanes, earthquakes, landslides, volcanic eruptions, wildfires, droughts, and extreme temperatures, with greater mitigation and resiliency needed to protect populations. This is complicated by the intensity and frequency of these events, revealing a growing threat to the most at-risk populations from highland to urban, rural, and coastal communities. The projections that climate change will cause more droughts, more frequently and intensely, especially in the Caribbean coupled with the growing food insecurity in the Northern Triangle of Central America offer a glimpse into the risk, hazards, and vulnerability analysis that are multifaceted and not always simple to resolve. Chapter 5 explores the history of collaboration, co-operation, and coordination within the Americas on transborder health issues as an important component of international affairs. This includes the contributions of vaccine diplomacy and scientific diplomacy, with new actors helping to shape public health diplomacy in contemporary times. This will show why greater transparency and sharing of information are important components of achieving public health security. In Chapter 6, I discuss how population health issues historically have been framed as humanitarian, social justice, or human rights concerns, with an increased emphasis on the securitization of public health challenges. This focus shows the intersection of public health and security with newly emerging and re-emerging infectious diseases in the Americas, heightened concerns about the increasing threat of antimicrobial resistance, and the consequences of biosecurity and biosafety associated with the naturally occurring, unintentional, or intentional spread of deadly pathogens. The conclusion will illustrate how the COVID-19 pandemic influences and is influenced by such broader relationships explored in the proceeding chapters on economic and political development, globalization, disaster and climate crisis, diplomacy, and security.

The challenges and humbling experiences I gained through field work have greatly influenced the way I perceive a complex public health puzzle with an inextricable relationship beyond the focus on health. Respectfully, I leave the medical issues to the subject area medical and health experts since these are an important piece of the puzzle, and beyond my knowledge or intent of this book.

In the text that follows, I will also include some of my experiences in the region of the Americas, where I first learned to use the zoom out lens, reset the focus beyond a simple health indicator, and respect insights even if they are "as far off as they seem." Howard Frumkin, fittingly stated, "complexity confuses, numbers numb, pictures persist, stories stick,"[8] to which I add, images illuminate. I attempt to balance this approach for the reader, as best as possible.

Notes

1 Marcos Cueto and Steven Palmer, *Medicine and Public Health in Latin America: A History*. (Cambridge: Cambridge University Press, 2015).
2 Pan American Health Organization, *Core Indictors 2019: Health Trends in the Americas* (Washington, DC: PAHO, 2019), 6.
3 Julio Frenk, José Luis Bobadilla, and Rafael Lozando, "The Epidemiological Transition in Latin America," *Notas de población* 22, no. 60 (1994): 79–101.
4 Julio Frenk et al., "Health Transition in Middle-Income Countries: New Challenges for Health Care," *Health Policy Planning* 4, no. 1 (1989): 29–39.
5 Alberto Barcelo et al., "The Cost of Diabetes in Latin America and the Caribbean in 2015: Evidence for Decision and Policy Makers, *Journal of Global Health* 7, (2017). doi:10.7189/jogh.07.020410. See also Organisation for Economic Co-operation and Development and The World Bank, *Health at a Glance: Latin America and the Caribbean 2020* (Paris: OECD Publishing, 2020), doi:10.1787/6089164f-en.
6 Food and Agriculture Organization of the United Nations, "United Nations Calls for Urgent Action to Curb the Rise in Hunger and Obesity in Latin America and the Caribbean," November 12, 2019, http://www.fao.org/news/story/en/item/1250781/icode/.
7 Ibid.
8 Howard Frumkin, "What Is Planetary Health and Why Now?" (Presentation, Planetary Health Seminar, Cambridge, MA: Harvard University, 2018).

1
PUBLIC HEALTH

Public health is about the spectrum of population health and health-related issues, and the collective actions to prevent, promote, maintain, and secure the well-being of peoples. It necessitates a greater appreciation of the determinants of health. It is those underlying factors that contribute to both good and bad public health outcomes. It was unfortunate that public health in the United States was viewed as a separate health care system of health departments that serve the poor, until more recently when the pandemic hit and public health became a household term.

Many Latin American countries chose a different path in response to a more collective health approach, with the rise in the social medicine movements during the 19th century. Western Europe had a great influence on Latin America's social policies to scrutinize economic inequalities, social class, and other structural factors associated with poor population health outcomes. At the same time, United States was providing education and training to health professionals in the region, and the Rockefeller Foundation and other regional organizations, such as the Pan American Sanitation Bureau, were helping to drive the population health policy agenda. The external influences in the late 1850s and early 1900s may be no different from what we see today, with powerful foundations driving the global to regional public health strategies.

Health to Public Health

Since the founding of the World Health Organization (WHO) in 1948, the uniformly accepted definition of health remains as, "the state of complete physical, mental, and social wellbeing and not merely the absence of disease or infirmity." Yet, still today, the focus remains on the physical assessments of disease

DOI: 10.4324/9781003007401-2

or illness. This traditional biomedical approach subjugates the important contributions of the political, economic, social, cultural, environmental, ecological, and technological factors in society and their impact on population health.

We talk about public health, yet the focus remains on medical solutions. The commitment to invest in the best public health practices and policies is based upon prevention, which remains difficult to motivate decision-makers to support when there are so many competing societal issues of importance. It is unfortunate, however, that public health has sparked limited interest, historically, until a crisis threatens the lives of decision-makers, economically, politically, or emotionally.

The challenge to invest in preventing something that may never happen is the public health battle cry. Striking the right balance to promote public health actions and social policy highlights an exigent path of prevention and protection, especially for at-risk populations. Prevention through such strategies as promoting seat belts, helmets, healthier diets, vaccination policies, mandatory quarantines, or reducing air pollution has led to contentious battles as forms of control versus protection, with no simple solutions. Is it the access to better technology, better education, higher incomes, improved infrastructure, or enforcement and sanctions that provides the best public health protection? It often depends upon where you sit that will influence your point of view. Investments in public health have paid off with great improvements throughout Latin America and the Caribbean, albeit not equally.

Clarity about public health was offered to me very early in my career. I had the opportunity to train and work in Latin America with Professor David Taplin, the head of University of Miami's Field Epidemiology Survey Team (FEST). He was a noted tropical disease microbiologist who studied infections and infestation of the skin and maintained that while such diseases may not appear to be a prioritized public health concern, they are a major drain on the health care delivery system with populations unnecessarily suffering. This approach provided a big picture view of public health and its inextricable relationship to poverty, environment, living conditions, lack of potable water and hygiene, as well as the structural determinants creating the political will of governments to invest in prevention. I saw it up close in my early field work in Colombia, Panama, Honduras, and Peru. What I also learned through such experiences is that relieving outbreaks of skin infestations and infections can build good relationships with communities since people may immediately feel better, sleep better, and concentrate more without the persistent itching and annoyance. This is where taking the time to understand how people feel matters. A Westernized assumption focuses its attention on what has been referred to as the real needs while we tend to overlook the felt needs. Real needs are based upon what we can measure, then quantify, and as such reveal how many doctors or nurses per population or hospital beds per population are needed. To be responsive we must draw our attention to such felt needs, that is what people feel they need. This requires a better balance of real and felt needs to improve health and well-being of a population.[1] Using a community-based participatory strategy has shown the benefit of gathering insights from the recipients of any community-driven health program. An example shared by a colleague shows as she was conducting a study in Colombia to determine the best location for a community health center, she found that people did not feel they needed a health center, and they could take a bus to a nearby location. Rather, they preferred a childcare center as a better investment. Listening to voices of the people in a community is a core component of public health actions. It does not matter if we are talking about mitigating a disease outbreak, or encouraging vaccinations, or promoting public health education to prevent or reduce obesity, high blood pressure, or heart disease.

In the early 1980s I was also fortunate to meet Dr. Carlos "Choclo" Monge, a Peruvian physician with a profound understanding of population health. One of his visits to Miami coincided with our team's preparation for a "pilot" field survey on the rates of skin infections and infestations in selected indigenous communities along the Ucayali River in Peru with travel to both tropical lowland Amazon and *altiplano* (high plain) regions.

While Taplin introduced me to the complexity of public health in real-world situations, Monge introduced me to the concept of human ecological niches as a measure of health beyond a biomedical reference. This was the ecological and cultural factors. Monge shared the example of how hemoglobin levels vary among groups living in tropical versus highlands regions. Hemoglobin is a known health indicator that measures the red blood cell count, which carries oxygen to the organs and tissues in the body. Low levels of hemoglobin will indicate anemia, a condition that makes one feel weak and tired. The normal level range was based upon a medical standard, since no one wanted to hire or keep someone employed if they seemed too weak to work. Therefore, in order to meet the determined medical requirement, workers at low altitude would give themselves iron to boost hemoglobin levels while high altitude workers would remove blood just to satisfy pre-determined standards.[2] Such measures were insufficient and revealed a much broader understanding of the ecology, environment, and culture concerning the study of population health.

Infrastructure and Public Health

Great improvements in public health infrastructure have been made in Latin America and the Caribbean, although 34 million are still using unimproved drinking water sources and 18 million have no access to sanitation services with one in ten living in rural areas across ten countries using open defecation.[3] Access to critical public health infrastructure and related health disparities has its roots in social and economic development, but political exigencies should not be excluded from the broader analysis. As stated in the introduction to this book, history has shown us how public health has significantly improved across industrialized nations such as England, Wales, and the United States in the early 1900s. This depended upon the political will to invest in better housing, potable water, sanitation, nutrition, and family planning. Controlling pests and vermin and promoting cleanliness with access to safe water and disposal of human waste and refuse have become the fundamental building blocks of public health.

With population shifts and fast urbanization, the United States learned important lessons in the early 1900s about the significance of public health along with the growth of cities, industrialization, and poverty. Pestilence and filth plagued the expanding cities until it became evident that health improvements rested upon the provision of improved infrastructure, better nutrition, improved working conditions, and the political will to encourage these investments. Nevertheless, post-WWII, the U.S. foreign assistance focused on a mixed bag of strategies to Latin America and the Caribbean versus the need for building and strengthening public health infrastructure. During the 1960s the emphasis was placed on vaccines and antibiotics as the investment in potable water, disposal of human waste and refuse, and appropriate protective housing was never fully realized equally throughout the region. A public health approach toward lifestyle changes shifted in the 1980s from infectious diseases to chronic disease prevention; yet, the burden of communicable diseases continued to disproportionately impact the poor.

Latin America and the Caribbean has made great progress in improving the access to safe water with variations within and across countries based upon urban and rural differences, as well as racial and ethnic populations. According to the Inter-American Development Bank's World Water Week Report 2019, 490 million people (69% of the population in the region) still lack appropriate sanitation and 80% of the industrial and residential wastewater is untreated, thereby increasing the risk to freshwater. Let's consider populations without access to safe water, sanitation, housing, and the relationship to public health. The example of a child with diarrhea shows how we think about the problem will influence how we respond. Applying a biomedical approach suggests we treat diarrhea with antibiotics if it is a bacterial infection or fluids to prevent dehydration. A behavioral approach seeks to educate mothers about how to reduce the risks at home and the necessity of handwashing, overall hygiene, and providing fluids. A broader sustainable consideration is to provide the necessary infrastructure as an investment in human development. The political and economic investments in public health address the structural barriers and highlight the inequities, imbalanced resource allocation, and power relations that continue to perpetuate poor health outcomes. This is where the state takes responsibility for the health and welfare of its people.

Poor infrastructure is also associated with childhood infestations from helminths (parasitic worms), which are endemic in many resource poor areas. Research by 2019 Nobel Prize for Economics, Esther Duflo and Abhijit Banerjee

(MIT's Abdul Latif Jameel Poverty Action Lab (JAPAL) and Michael Kramer (Harvard) shows greater educational outcomes and better school attendance with fewer absences due to illnesses through simple deworming treatments. Their evidence-based research documents better educational performance from deworming compared to giving children books. Using rigorous scientific methods, such as what is used in clinical drug trials, researchers were able to place science squarely into the nexus of public health and development, with focus on alleviating poverty. However, the question arises, could deworming children serve as band aid approach to much deeper problems? Would it not be better to provide the improved infrastructure and reduce the threat of re-infestations? The simple answer is yes.

The lack of a sound public health infrastructure provides a happy home to microbes and disease vectors, which may place the most vulnerable at risk for illness, disease, and injury. Another example is the case study of Mexico's *Piso Firme* (Solid Foundation) initiated in 2000 to lessen parasitic infections and improve child health. The government's commitment to install cement floors in homes where previous dirt floors existed resulted in 20% less parasitic infestations, almost 30% fewer cases of diarrhea, and 20% less cases of anemia along with the improved cognition of children. The unexpected outcomes also revealed that mother's depression decreased by 12.5% and perceived stress by 10.4%.[4] This evidence supports investments in housing, coupled with a targeted engineering approach to replace dirt floors with cement will reduce parasitic infestations with a range of other health-promoting benefits for a family.

Terms

Epidemiology is the science of public health. It is centered on the provision of evidence-based research to study population health. The most noted historical example is the classic field epidemiological work by John Snow in 1854 that identified the source of a cholera outbreak from the Thames River in London. Recognized as the father of epidemiology, Snow reasoned that if he removed the handle from the Broad Street pump the spread of cholera would cease since this contaminated water was the point of entry into a community. However, it was the engineering of a fully integrated sewer system in the late 19th century led by Joseph Bazalgette that mitigated any future major outbreaks of cholera again in London. Thus, it takes a multidisciplinary team to successfully respond to public health challenges.

Contrary to what is often assumed, epidemiology is not the study of epi-demics. It is the study of the distribution and spread of disease, illness, injury, or death within a population. It is a Latin term whereby the *epi* (upon) *demos* (the people) *logos* (to study) provides the scientific basis for implementing public health interventions. It employs a triangular approach to investigate people, place, and time, considering how the host, agent, and environment interact.

Epidemiologic studies were first based upon the study of infectious diseases, to identify who was getting infected, what caused the disease, and where it was occurring to mitigate the spread of an infectious agent. Today epidemiology is widely used to exercise the best practices to reduce population risk from a communicable or noncommunicable disease, mental health, injuries, and violence.

For example, gender violence is an important public health issue. In 2017, the United Nations Development Report ranked Latin America number one in the world for reported cases of sexual violence against women. Using epidemiologic methods to identify the victims and perpetrators, weapons used, and location of such acts helps communities to implement actions to prevent and mitigate future life-threatening incidents. Such data provide insights into the at-risk population at risk, types of injuries anticipated or deaths due to the weapons used, and the likelihood of an event occurring at a residence, workplace, or other locations. In Central America, 66% of the women killed were due to femicide, a more recent category of homicide where 15 countries in Latin America identify it as a crime today. Gender inequality is an important factor to consider as are other social issues as underlying factors of such violence. Even with the growing scientific evidence, policies are not uniformly carried out across the region, and it is likely underreported. An Oxfam July 2018 study, *Enough – Together We Can End Violence Against Girls And Women*, showed the trends and comparative analysis of gender-based violence in Bolivia, Colombia, Cuba, Dominican Republic, El Salvador, Guatemala, Honduras, and Nicaragua. Interviews with 20–25-year-old participants showed how 56% men and 48% women reported having a friend who was a victim of male violence in the past year, where 84% of both men and women felt gender violence against women was the outcome of inequalities and 67% reported that they deemed this a responsibility of their government.[5] Studying violence as a public health issue exemplifies a broader analysis of the risks of injuries, disabilities, and deaths, thereby targeting women throughout the region with greater investments in the social and structural determinants of gender-based violence.

We hear the echoing of eradication efforts to fight poverty, world hunger, disease, or violence. These lofty goals may never be fully realized. However, implementing strategies to reduce the impact on populations' welfare offers a positive role for public health actions with clear objectives to reduce the impact on morbidity and mortality. Such studies can be scaled up and adapted as appropriate for a targeted population.

The embellishment of the term eradicate has an important meaning in public health. The confusion on terms of controlling, eliminating, and eradicating disease continues. It is useful to clarify terms since they are often used as colloquial expressions and not always helpful to understanding public health. Controlling a disease means reducing old and new cases and deaths to a locally acceptable level. This takes place through active interventions, community engagement, and sustainable policies to protect populations. I collaborated on a community-based scabies project from 1986 to 1990 in Guna Yala, Panama among the Guna Indians. Scabies is a tiny mite that borrows under the skin causing itching and often secondary infections due to the incessant scratching. Scabies was brought to the island communities in the 1970s and spread easily due to the living conditions, close contact, and lack of potable water. The persistent itching from scabies causes a disruption in life from sleeping, working, or studying. In this collaborative effort to control the infestation, community leaders, local population, ministry of health, and community health workers collectively identified, treated, managed, and maintained ongoing surveillance. A prevalence of 33%, of which 25% were very severe cases of scabies infestations, was reduced to less than 2% severe cases. This was a manageable level for local community control. As indicated above, this was not the highest priority at first, but it soon became one with the halt to annoying itching and willingness of the population to engage in further health-promoting initiatives. I will expand upon this in Chapter 5 to exemplify the important intersection of diplomacy and public health.

Eliminating a disease means reducing all new cases to zero at the national or regional level with continuing surveillance and tracking to prevent new cases. Latin America and the Caribbean have been free of polio for 26 years. In 1975, the Pan American Health Organization (PAHO) reported 6,000 children inflicted with paralytic polio; however, through a continuous public health vaccination program by 1994 the region eliminated polio and the last case was reported in a child from highland Peru. With hopes to eradicate polio the challenge still remains in Nigeria, Afghanistan, and Pakistan. In Latin America and the Caribbean region, the elimination of rubella, known as German measles or three-day measles, and congenital rubella was announced in 2015.

The eradication of a disease means it is permanently removed from anywhere in the world and no further interventions are necessary. To date, the only known human disease to ever be eradicated is smallpox. The last known case in the Americas was found in 1971 in Brazil and the last case in the world in 1977 in Somalia. The success depended greatly on the accessibility to a global vaccine program and the robust public health efforts that engaged communities and will be explored further in Chapter 3 on globalization and public health.

Another term that is often overlooked is extinction. This signifies that an infectious agent causing a disease no longer exists anywhere. Smallpox virus does not exist in nature, but viral stocks do remain in laboratories in both the United States and Russia. The controversy of keeping stockpiles of this viral agent or destroying them has been especially important in the United States since the post-9/11 attack was followed weeks later with a bioterrorist act using anthrax.

Public health problems are complex, multidimensional, fluid social issues, and require multiple sectors beyond the medical and health fields. Such challenges as poverty, malnutrition and food insecurity, obesity, or climate change are considered wicked issues that disproportionately impact the health of vulnerable populations. The term wicked problem was first used in the 1970s for community planning and social policies. It challenged the simplistic approach to the questions, answers, solutions, and proposed policies driving decision making.[6] By embracing the concept of wicked problems we accept that a broader collaboration with public and private partnerships, community participation, strong leadership, and the political will to address public health, safety, and security is necessary. However, along with the diverse stakeholders' perspectives are many ways to approach an issue with different solutions.[7] Key stakeholders often agree on the goals for such things as eliminating poverty or reducing and improving nutritional outcomes; the disagreement arises from the competing perspectives and consequent strategies to achieve a desired goal. Thus, different perceptions about the underlying causes of community health problem will influence different strategies. Such interventions could collide, rather than converge to foster cooperation. This may bring about unintended consequences such as violating human rights; if good, rigorous evaluations of the programs or policies are not well monitored along the way. For example, during the early research and treatment for HIV/AIDS, where the Caribbean region reported the second highest rates in the world, there were unintended outcomes of further stigmatizing already marginalized populations. This demands greater attention to the social and societal determinants of public health in response to wicked issues and solution. There are many ways to study population health. This includes the determinants of health related to biological or heredity factors; access to healthcare services and technology; lifestyle and behaviors; environment; and social, cultural, political, and economic factors. It is these social and societal determinants that provide a clearer understanding of the inequalities and health inequities in Latin America and the Caribbean.

Social Determinants of Health

Social determinants of health (SDoH) have become the guiding principles of public health practice. The WHO/PAHO defines SDoH as "the conditions in which people are born, grow, work, live, and age, and the wider set of forces and systems sharing the conditions of daily life." These include a range of political, economic, social, cultural, environmental, and ecological, to technological considerations. In early 1990, Mexico's National Solidarity Program set the platform for policies to reduce poverty and target health inequalities. Mexico has invested greatly into SDoH. The most rigorously evaluated program was the conditional cash transfer (CCT) first initiated in 1997 and the successful social welfare programs such as Seguro Popular 2007, which highlighted Mexico's commitment to improving health outcomes beyond the single focus of the health sector. Argentina, Brazil, and Chile have all included SDoH into their national governmental structures as part of their strategy. The Rio Political Declaration on Social Determinants of Health was adopted during the

WHO World Conference on Social Determinants of Health in 2011 to support a global commitment to reduce health inequities and create the political will to promote the implementation of SDoH at the country level with appropriate targeted strategies within each country. In Latin America SDoH were also included in the Ministers of Health 2010–2015 Plan of Action and the PAHO's 2014–2019 Strategic Plan with ongoing evaluations.

History of Public Health and Social Determinants

I do not intend to provide a comprehensive historical analysis of public health in the region. I refer the reader to the excellent work by Cueto and Palmer.[8] The purpose is to show the trajectory of a population health paradigm, and how it has influenced research, practice, and public policies in Latin America and the Caribbean through examples. I have selected examples to reinforce why it is necessary to go beyond the measure of a health indicator to understand population health outcomes. This includes the interconnectedness of internal and external influences on population health associated with the wider concerns of development, globalization, disasters and climate crisis, diplomacy, and security.

Historically, the dominant paradigm for public health rested upon the assumption that economic growth would miraculously trickle down to improve health conditions for all. Latin America saw the realities of such failed policies bringing the shift toward social medicine and a collective health movement in the 1970s. This conveyed the importance of using the analytical tools of social science in response to public health and the rise of contemporary social medicine movement in Latin America.

The social medicine movement in Latin America was also greatly influenced by the research, teachings, and laws of Europe, in which social determinants were identified as the key factors in understanding poor population outcomes. The United Kingdom's 1980 Black Report studied class-based health patterns and mortality associated with the social and economic determinants. It also placed the spotlight on the increasing inequalities in mortality. While not first accepted by the Conservative Party since it was deemed as too costly, later review on the inequalities conducted through the Acheson Report provided a new blueprint to reduce health inequalities in the United Kingdom by describing public health as the collective actions to maintain and sustain population-centered approaches for health improvements. The Acheson Report defined what remains as the widely accepted definition of public health as, "the art and science of preventing disease, promoting health, and prolonging life through organized efforts of society."[9] Furthermore, Western Europe's Whitehall studies on inequalities in health along with Sir Michael Marmot's pivotal work on the SDoH gave further support for the social gradient and public health studies. History reveals how the political activities during the social and political reform movements in Europe, the Spanish Civil War (1936–1939), along with Latin America's progressive approach to health and medicine in the early 20th century, helped shape public health across the region.

Earlier work from the 17th-century London's Bill of Mortality by Graunt and Perry and the Poor Laws of 19th century had already explored the social and economic relationship of health, illness, and disease. The 1800s became an active time for enlightenment of public health; in 1842, Edwin Chadwick showed the relationship between poor sanitation, poverty, and disease. The 19th-century scientist and politicians offered keen insight into the poor health conditions in England. Edwin Chadwick (1800–1890), one of the key architects of The Poor Law Act of 1834, reasoned that the unsanitary conditions of the impoverished people were a key factor in poor health and disease outcomes. He argued that improving the social living conditions would result in a healthier and more productive society. Therefore, improving public health would be a smart preventive investment for long-term economic development. The key investments included safe water, improved drainage and provision for sewers, and the collection of refuse. These remain the fundamental building blocks of public health protection.

It was the influence by Rudolf Virchow (1821–1902), respected German pathologist, often referred to as the father of social medicine, that requires more attention as it relates to Latin America and the Caribbean. Virchow fought for social reforms and political leadership to promote societal changes to improve health. One of his most notable contributions to public health occurred in 1848 when he studied the typhus outbreak in Prussia.[10] He detailed how the poor living conditions and government's failure to address such inadequate social conditions were the underlying causes of the outbreak. This seminal work contributed to developing anthropology as an important scientific discipline and shining a light on medicine, social sciences, and political actions. His notable quote, "medicine is social science, and politics is nothing else but medicine on a large scale," suggests a demand for transdisciplinary study and practice. This is important to what has taken place in Latin America, where a structural preventive approach became the foundation of social medicine, which was not necessarily achieved equally throughout the region. Virchow's teaching had a great influence on Chile, and specifically on then medical student Salvador Allende, often considered the father of the 20th-century social medicine movement in Latin America. We cannot overlook the relationship to political systems in Latin American countries where repressive regimes and military dictatorships forced changes in the collective public health shifts.

The advocacy for structural changes to improve health outcomes provided a new home for social medicine in many Latin American countries. Chile's social medicine movement in 1918 coincided with the strikes for better working conditions. Salvador Allende's call to improve social and economic conditions as factors in poor health influenced the wider social movements in Cuba, Brazil,

Ecuador, Mexico, and Nicaragua, which all brought significant attention to population health and human welfare in the region. Social medicine in Latin America considered social class in relation to economic production versus the approach of public health used in the United States.[11] While at this time the United States focused on medical care and treatments, and less on prevention, many Latin American countries explored the European path that would attend to the underlying social and societal determinants of health. This was not an easy path.

Salvador Allende's 1939 book on social medicine, *La Realidad Médico-Social Chilena* (The Chilean Socio-Medical Reality) argued that ill health and diseases were caused by the poor social and economic conditions. He directed his attention to the structural factors that exacerbated poverty, and how the poor working conditions contributed to emotional and occupational-related diseases, maternal and infant mortality, tuberculosis, and sexually transmitted diseases.[12] The attention to mental health showed his enlightened perspective into public health challenges still facing Latin American society and culture today.

Before his election as president in 1970, Salvador Allende was a pathologist, minister of health, and the architect of the first national health service for Latin America. Later as a senator he exposed the inextricable relationship of social justice, social reforms, and social medicine proposing radical structural changes for a new approach to population health. His controversial approach probed deeper into the structural inequities, access to resources, and power, which were not welcomed by all. It was the 1973 military coup, and the death of Allende, which set forth a new era of public health in Chile coinciding with the growth of neoliberal policies in the 1980s This focused on market-driven approaches of competitiveness with cost-effectiveness and cost efficiency in health care systems in the region and less on public health and spread throughout the region.

Cuba's Public Health

Earlier transitions in the Caribbean country of Cuba provide another point of view about the history of public health in the region. The 1959 Cuban Revolution, led by Fidel Castro, made health care a virtue of socialism operating a Marxist-Leninist approach to the formation of one government rule of the Cuban Communist Party. The Cuban health care system, recognized for its unified, decentralized, and comprehensive approach defined in a social political system, has also been equally criticized for existing as a form of social control. *"La salud es derecho para todos y la responsabilidad del Estado"* (health is a right for all and the responsibility of the State, according to the Cuban Ministry of Public Health). Fidel Castro made Cuba's good health indicators "the true test of government efficacy and the health of the individual a symbol of the health of the 'body politic'," as described by Feinsilver in her book, *Healing the Masses*.[13] Yet, Cuba's impressive health indicators of lower infant mortality and higher life expectancy were documented well before the arrival of Castro's regime with the country's earlier investments in public health infrastructure and tropical disease research. Cuba's world recognized Pedro Kouri Institute of Tropical Medicine (PKI) was founded at the University of Havana in 1937 and is known for its excellence in research on parasitic diseases such as malaria. While this institute lost its leadership after the death of Pedro Kouri in 1964, in 1979 Fidel Castro moved PKI to the Ministry of Health and expanded it to include other infectious disease research, education, and training as well as public health interventions.

Since the revolution, Cuba is often promoted as a public health model for the world. Based upon what we know, can public health be fully realized without a respect for human rights? My question is controversial.

Simply stated, human rights are core international values that are fundamental to public health. The argument that Cuba's evidence-based research supports excellent health status indicators necessarily raises more questions. We recognize that water systems, sewage, housing, waste disposal, and good nutrition are all basic building blocks for a sound public health system and essential to good health outcomes. The neglected and failing water, sewage, garbage, and housing systems have been documented in Cuba, with corroding and leaking water pipes, lack of garbage collection, spillage of sewage, and dilapidated insufficient housing along with the country's vulnerability to disasters and climate change presenting great health challenges for Cuba.

During the 1980s, Cuba's commitment to community-based health became the model for primary health care and was highly regarded by many practitioners, scientists, and leaders throughout the globe. I first read an analysis questioning if Cuba's health care system was a model of service or a form of social control that raised important questions.[14] Then, during the mid-1990s a representative of the Cuban Ministry of Health presented a paper at an international public health conference in Washington, DC. At the conclusion I asked the speaker and wider audience if they understood the depth of distrust and fiery anger against Fidel Castro and the Cuban regime by many Cuban Americans in Miami. Shortly after, Wayne Smith, a former head of the US Interest Section in Cuba, offered a trip for Cuban Americans in South Florida to have an up-close look at the public health situation in Cuba. I reached out to colleagues and others from the community with encouragement and a promise that their participation as a Cuban American would not be disclosed. Despite an Alpha 66 threat prior to departure on a chartered flight, and an empty promise of anonymity, I had to question both sides of the continuing debate. The aggressive acts from the Alpha 66 anti-Castro paramilitary group in Miami against the deception of the Cuban government created the academic and practical discussion of idealism versus realism of public health systems. After apologizing to those who did not want their names or faces exposed, I reflected upon the health data that were presented, when people didn't have access to sufficient food, reliable safe water, soap, toilet paper, or adequate garbage collection? Weren't these the building block requirements for public health?

The zenith of Cuba's "special period" from 1991 to 1993 corresponded with the optic neuropathy epidemic. We learned that damage to the eyes was due to the lack of sufficient vitamins and a weakened society that coincided with the fall of the former Soviet Republic and Cuba's dependency for financial support. How could this happen if public health was the government's priority? I read with great interest Pedro Coutlin-Churchman's journal article on *Cuban Epidemic Neuropathy: A Glimpse from Inside a Totalitarian Disease*[15] in which he reminds us that even with a universal health care approach, the government controlled all food and markets that contributed to the suffering of its own people.

Public health investment includes protecting human rights. This means not restricting health professionals from speaking out for releasing public health data about a disease outbreak that the government wants to keep as a state secret. In 1997 Dr. Dessy Mendoza was jailed in Cuba for talking to a Miami radio station about the outbreak of dengue hemorrhagic fever on the island. This also means sharing timely health data and not deny or be forced to concede when outbreaks are exposed through laboratory confirmation of travelers returning to their home countries. In interviews I learned that well-planned public health actions to fight vector- and water-borne diseases, such as dengue and cholera, were aggressively implemented more recently. Sadly, health professionals were directed to euphemistically use the terms of febrile illnesses for dengue fever and gastrointestinal upsets for cholera, in contradiction to public health transparency and empowering people with the truth.

Cuban government's delay to share official public health data in a timely manner is not a new issue. This epidemiologic silence is most disturbing because Cuba has a top notched health surveillance system. In May 2017, Dr. Jason Harris, Associate Professor of Pediatrics at Harvard Medical School in an interview with *Drug Development & Discovery Magazine*, remarked that while the Cuban government may not report cases, "there continue to be sporadic cases of cholera in travelers from Cuba,"[16] further revealing a gap in the protection of citizens and tourist. This occurred at the same time Cuba received a top 2017 WHO recognition[17] for their support to international health emergencies such as their response to Ebola and other South-South collaborations. Cuba is highly recognized for their medical diplomacy outreach to help resource poor countries fill gaps in medical care, combat outbreaks, or respond to pandemics. Today we take a note of their important contributions to medical diplomacy for COVID-19.

Nevertheless, at home the Cuban government's repression of rights continues. According to Human Rights Watch (2017)[18] from January to August 2016 there were 7,900 reports of arbitrary detention in Cuba, showing an increase in such detentions in recent years along with other repressive actions. State sovereignty allows for such internal actions, and yet no national or international state or non-state actors seem to be able to change the conversation, not even when the disturbing graphic depictions of Cuban police forces dragging and jailing members of the women's human rights group, *Damas de Blanco*, dissidents, or the jailing of independent journalists for reporting the news is shared through traditional or social media. But soon after, unfortunately, the emotional reaction subsides. There are so many other competing global issues. Or is it that we remain silent in a noticeable attention deficient disorder world where one big event dominates the 24-hour news cycle until the next event arrives driving a fickle response? Has this become our 21st-century style of population indifference? I suggest, indifference is a powerful word and exposes the perplexity of broad-based problems where public health and human rights intersect.

We can no longer be indifferent to the human rights violation and then step up to admire a country for its promotion of public health and primary health care. This is a compelling contradiction. Cuba is clearly not the only country with continuing human rights violations; however, Cuba is one known violator we are willing to overlook the other way to promote the accolades of a free health care system, whether we question this or not. The case of Cuba and public health is intriguing and prompts a discussion of whether social justice and human rights are necessary components of public health. Cuba remains an enigma, which I will explore further in later chapters with the intent to create greater discussion.

Public Health Regional Focus

It was the outcome of a 1902 meeting in Mexico when the transition of the Pan American Sanitation Board to the PAHO emerged with the purpose to find a balance in regional trade of goods that would protect and secure the economic well-being of countries with safe public health practices. The enactment of the PAHO in Washington, DC came to fruition in December 1902 with ten countries in attendance. It is noteworthy that the PAHO was well established before the creation of the United Nations specialized health agency, the WHO in 1948. With headquarters in Geneva, Switzerland the WHO has six regional offices in Africa, the Americas (PAHO), Southeast Asia, Europe, Eastern Mediterranean, and West Pacific.

The PAHO headquarters remain in Washington, DC with 28 country offices spread throughout the region and three specialized centers to promote health, provide technical assistance, and facilitate evidence-based research for decision making. The main governing body of PAHO meets every five years for member states to address policies and elect a new director. Today a director can serve only two consecutive terms. From 1902 to 1959 the male leadership was a representative from the United States, while in the past 61 years leaders have come from countries throughout Latin America and the Caribbean. It

TABLE 1.1 World Health Organization Regional Offices and PAHO Members

World Health Organization	Geneva, Switzerland	Total Member States
Africa	Brazzaville, Congo	47 member states
Americas (OPS)-PAHO	**Washington, DC**	**35 members states**
Southeast Asia	New Delhi, India	11 member states
Europe	Copenhagen, Denmark	52 member states
Eastern Mediterranean	Cairo, Egypt	22 member states
West Pacific	Manila, Philippines	28 member states

Sources: World Health Organization and Pan American Health Organization.

TABLE 1.2 Pan American Health Organization (PAHO) Member States and
Chronology of Admission[a]

Country	Month/Year
United States	March 1925
Cuba	June 1925
Nicaragua	December 1925
El Salvador	May 1926
Haiti	June 1926
Peru	November 1926
Costa Rica	December 1926
Uruguay	December 1928
Mexico	March 1929
Panama	March 1929
Bolivia	March 1929
Brazil	October 1929
Chile	October 1929
Dominican Republic	November 1929
Ecuador	September 1930
Venezuela	March 1933
Guatemala	May 1933
Colombia	June 1933
Argentina	September 1937
Paraguay	June 1939
Honduras	January 1957
Jamaica	August 1962
Trinidad and Tobago	September 1963
Barbados	October 1967
Guyana	October 1967
Canada	September 1971
Bahamas	October 1974
Suriname	September 1976
Granada	September 1977
St. Lucia	September 1980
Dominica	September 1981

(Continued)

Country	Month/Year
St. Vincent and the Grenadines	September 1981
Antigua and Barbuda	September 1982
Belize	September 1982
St. Kitts and Nevis	September 1984

Source: Pan American Health Organization.
[a]   Associate Members of the PAHO: Puerto Rico September 1992 and Aruba, Curacao, and Sint Maarten all joined in September 2012.

took one century for the last two directors to become the first women leaders, Dr. Mirta Roses Períago from Argentina and current director, Dr. Carisa F. Etienne from the Caribbean island of Dominica (Tables 1.1 and 1.2).

Early History and the International Health Sanitary Conferences

During the 1800s, the epidemics of plague, cholera, and yellow fever required greater regional cooperation to control the spread of diseases. By the 1880s, after multiple rounds of the International Sanitary Conferences in the Americas, especially with expanding port cities, new sanitary agreements and health regulations related to regional trade between Brazil, Nicaragua, Peru, United States, and Venezuela came to fruition. The early concern that the International Health Sanitary Conferences were more about economic growth and political power than they were about science[19] and public health reverberates today.

Yellow fever (YF) has a long history with many outbreaks throughout the world and provides one of the best examples of regional public health perils. YF is a virus caused by the *aedes aegypti* mosquito and the same mosquito that causes dengue, chikungunya, and Zika. Currently, the only safe and effective vaccine exists for the prevention of YF. YF was likely introduced in Cuba from the Spanish colony in Yucatan, Mexico in 1648, with low levels of transmission and slow decline. However, further evidence documents that it was likely re-introduced into Cuba by infected prisoners from Vera Cruz sent to Havana to construct buildings in 1751.[20] The broader understanding of public health to include the environment, sanitary conditions, economic trade, and political conflict was already underway. In 1879 it was reported that "The Gulf ports, no doubt, with their handicaps of semi-tropical climate and of traditional indifference to sanitation, will remain open to its ravages so long as trade relations are maintained with such plague-breeding hotbeds as Havana and Vera Cruz."[21]

The history of the YF epidemic portrays the dual battle of disease and conflict during the Spanish-American War of 1898. While malaria was controlled with the use of quinine, at that time there was no known treatment for the raging epidemic of YF. Combat deaths were not in comparison to the thousands of more dying from the wrath of YF. Throughout history, militaries and wars have been major conduits for the spread of disease. More soldiers died from the 1918–1919 influenza pandemic than on the battlefield during World War I. Mosquitoes travel by easy hitchhiking a ride on boats and ships and sneak across borders as an undocumented, unwelcomed passenger. Therefore, the prevention, surveillance, detection, and response in early public health efforts in the region remain today. This requires multisectoral cooperation for collective action.

The completion of the Panama Canal would not have been successful without the collaboration between Cuba, Panama, and the United States. The French began the construction of the Panama Canal in 1881 which was deterred by the merciless mosquitoes that caused Frenchmen to die from yellow fever and malaria. Ultimately, the French were forced to abandon their labors, and in 1904 the United States took over to finally complete the canal in 1914. The construction of the Panama Canal is an excellent example of the intersection of public health, development, globalization, and regional cooperation as the art and science of health diplomacy and security which exemplifies the organization of the chapters in this book. It must begin by identifying the public health issues from distinct perspectives.

Reflections from the Field: Public Health – Traditional versus Western Medicine

Culture shapes how populations identify, define, and respond to health, illnesses, and diseases. This includes the beliefs, knowledge, morals, laws, and customs within the context of one's society. There has been a great deal written about the traditional health practice and their contributions to the physical, mental, and social well-being throughout Latin America and the Caribbean. My curiosity was prompted in early 1980s when a pruritic rash broke out across my chest. It occurred three days before I was traveling to South America for field work in Colombia and Peru. My health care provider prescribed hydrocortisone, a steroidal anti-inflammatory and anti-itch cream suggesting it was possibly an adverse reaction to the Hepatitis B vaccine I received a day prior. It was never confirmed that the rash was a reaction to the vaccine. I arrived in Colombia with little improvement after three days of applying the topical treatment. I was introduced to a *curandero* (traditional healer), residing in outskirts of Bogota. I thought, as long as I did not have to ingest anything, and just apply to my skin, maybe the herbs and plants would reduce the itching and redness. He prepared a poultice that included a mixture of plants and roots, referring to one of them a *lunaria*, a moon-shaped plant that documented medicinal use as far back as the 1500s. He placed the poultice across my chest and showed me how to prepare and apply it for the next two days. After the first application I felt a distinct improvement and by day two the redness and itching were both gone. While this was purely an anecdotal account and offered no scientific-based research to support its efficacy, it was my first experience with traditional health practices that elicited my curious exploration of using herbs, plants, and roots.

Two years after that experience I was in the Central Eastern portion of the Amazon, in Pucallpa, Peru, where I learned about the Shipibo Indian's beliefs and use of traditional medicine. I was especially intrigued by the detailed sketched books of different plants and their intended use. The population lacked access to modern medicines while their strong beliefs in the healing powers of their lush vegetation and use of their land remained rooted into their day-to-day medicinal practices. The power of the land to produce plants to protect as well as to heal was based upon the belief to live in harmony with one's land. Sounded to me that this was getting to the root of the meaning of public health.

In my search for more information, I came across Nicole Maxwell's *Witch-doctor's Apprentice* written in 1961,[22] a fascinating book about her medicinal plant research in South America that began in the 1940s. Born in 1902 from a wealthy California oil family, Maxwell trained as a biologist at Harvard, who later fled a failing marriage to visit friends in South America. She appeared to be an unlikely explorer to travel deep into the jungles in search of natural medicines. Her interest in the science of the healing plants happened by chance when she received a deep machete wound while trekking through the Amazon. Her guide immediately scooped up a reddish tree sap which he told her to drink to stop the bleeding. By her account, and to her surprise, the bleeding stopped quickly and left her without scarring. This aroused her curiosity of the healing power plants used among the indigenous populations throughout South America, where she continued to study hundreds of different species throughout her life as she built strong relationships, especially among Indigenous women. In Iquitos, Peru she learned about the secret of *piri-piri*, a natural contraceptive plant. Fascinated by its potential, Maxwell reached out to U.S. pharmaceutical company and received financial support to study such medicinal plants. Unfortunately, the company was never really interested in her pursuit for scientific research. To her dismay, it was more about the publicity to profile a woman traveling through the jungle alone than it was about the medicinal value of plants. Maxwell continued her work to study nature's pharmacopeia and build strong relationships with Indigenous women. In an interview with the *Washington Post* in 1983, Maxwell shared her frustration with the lack of interest and concern that the acculturation process and growth of modern civilization will lose sight of the benefit of nature's healing agents.[23] She died at the age of 92, so possibly her lifelong commitment to nature's healing power was her path to longevity.

Well-known modern drugs today have their origin in trees, leaves, seeds, roots, and bark. In 1785 the discovery of the chemical digitoxin was found in the foxglove plant, also known as *digitalis purpurea*, and used in the treatment of heart disease. In the 1880s a German scientist found that the willow tree contained acetylsalicylic acid, the derivative of what we know today as aspirin. One of the most important contributions to public health in the tropics was the identification of quinine found in the *chinchona* tree and referred to as fever bark used to treat malaria. It is also recognized in the literature as Jesuit's bark since it was used by Jesuit missionaries in Peru dating back to the 1600s. Today, we are more familiar with a synthetic form to treat malaria called chloroquine and hydroxychloroquine. It is also known as the controversial drug for COVID-19. Hydroxychloroquine was promoted by Brazil's President, Jair Bolsonaro, along with other leaders, such as President Donald Trump of the United States, even though no rigorous studies to support the safety and efficacy for this treatment were available.

Earlier history documents the exploitation of forests and extraction of this highly sought-after magic bark for malaria, as the Spanish controlled the Andes region. Pharmaceutical companies had limited interest in developing a drug for malaria since it mostly inflicted the poor who could not afford to pay for treatment. That changed with populations movements and the emergence and re-emergence of the mosquito carrying the parasite. We note little difference today with industry balancing their profits with philanthropy. It comes as no surprise that there is more financial investment in research and development for chronic diseases impacting both rich and poor nations, with aggressive strategies to market to populations that can pay for costly new drugs.

The relationship between traditional and Western health practices in Latin America and the Caribbean is not necessarily a seamless one. Beliefs and healing practices have a long history of influencing public health practices in the region from Amerindian, Afro-Caribbean, Afro-Latin American, and Luso-Hispanic populations. In the late 1970s the WHO identified ways to view the existing relationships as parallel, tolerant, or integrated health care systems. This was associated with where one lived, not necessarily the country, but the topography and ecosystem from forest, tropical, temperate across highland to lowland communities where similar and dissimilar cultural practices and interpretations were observed with the availability and access to alternative options beyond plants, seeds, trees, roots, sand, and rocks. Probably one of the most recognized example of a fully integrated health delivery system is in China, with its widely accepted use of modern medicines complemented with traditional Chinese medicine interventions such as herbal remedies achieving the ying-yang balance of a healthy life. On the opposite spectrum, the United States functioned as parallel systems, until more recently, a transition to more tolerant approaches of selected alternative health care practices as some become covered by health insurance.

According to anthropologist, George Foster, the history of traditional humoral beliefs and practices, theory of hot-cold balance, has also been documented in Peru in the 1870s with old world origins.[24] This plays an important role in both historical and contemporary times in Latin America and is based upon the belief that a disruption of the human balance will cause an illness requiring therapies *frio* (cold) therapies for *caliente* (hot) illnesses.

Integrating traditional health practices within Western health care systems is not well understood. One misrepresentation frequently reported in the literature is the use of traditional health practices within the Western health care system among the Guna Indians, an indigenous population in an archipelago on the northeast coast of Panama. It is stated that both practices have been fully integrated into a health care delivery system for prevention and treatment. Though the Ministry of Health provides modern medicines, vaccines, and valuable health information, people still depend upon their local healers for both prevention and therapeutics. This takes place while the patient-provider in the Western system and the patient-healer in the traditional system never seem to interact. To be a fully integrated health care system, a best practice would be to have all providers collaborate or share information about a patient's health treatment. This has to do with culture, acceptance, and trust. Most of the writings about the curing practices of the Guna Indians are presented by anthropologists, with careful attention to the different levels, types, and methods used for healing. Over the decades, I have worked and lived among the Guna Indians and observed how a tolerant, yet parallel health care system co-exists within communities. While the elders show great trust for their local healers, and many old and young seeking help from a special healer may travel from other villages, and when accessible they will also use the allopathic Western medical system. Guna healing practices are performed in a private residences or in a healer's home, away from other patients. Yes, they co-exist, but I question the integration into a preventive or curative system. In 2015, some local healers tried to co-locate their services and provide a single site to care for traveling patients rather than use the healer's personal home. This was a great idea conceptualized by the aging healers, but it never came to fruition and since that time two healers have died.

In 2011, I arrived with a group of students to a remote Guna village with no electricity, internet, or computer services for a global public health and development field-based course. One of the healers, Eleuterio Adams, whom I have known for many years, asked if we could document his practices to include photographs and types of treatments. A group of students eagerly volunteered for the project, and a personal book on healing secrets was delivered to him later that year. As in most community health projects, this was made possible through a level of trust, and with a clear purpose to record his practices to pass down to future generations.

Eleuterio also encouraged positive health through the ritual bathing of herbs with special attention and protection to the head. This is a way of life. One such treatment ritual is used to open the mind and make a student feel more prepared to learn. As part of the educational experience, Rachel Libby, who had traveled to the community the prior year as a student and this time as my teaching assistant, was studying for the medical college admissions test and eager to partake in the bathing ritual for ten days. She was joined by Eleuterio's daughter, who was preparing to leave the island to study in the city. Rachel enjoyed the herbal bathing, which she described as relaxing, refreshing, and motivational. As she says, "It must have worked since I tested well," and today she is a practicing emergency room physician. Libby's subjective experience is a reminder of the historical to modern-day power of herbal bathing as hygienic, medicinal, and intentionally relaxing (Figure 1.1).

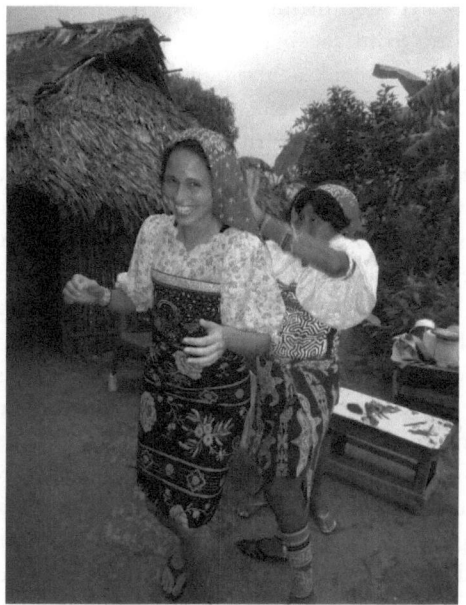

FIGURE 1.1 Rachel Libby, Post- Herbal Bathing Ritual, June 2011. By author.

During another field course learning opportunity, a great lesson was taught to the university students about the functioning of different health care systems among the Guna people. One of the most noted *sahilas* (chiefs) since the 1970s, Gonzalo Salcedo, was also known for his specialty as a bone healer and incorporating handpicked remedies collected from the mountains. Each healer has a connection to the land as they collect the plants, roots, trees, and sedimentary rocks for a treatment plan. Many healers use an additional chanting ceremony to promote physical, social, and spiritual curing practices. Again, this is a holistic approach to health as it was intended to be, where the physical, mental, and social well-being co-exists and emphasizes why it is important to preserve indigenous territories.

Gonzalo worked on the leg to encourage healing and applied a curative poultice of herbs and roots and wrapped the leg to facilitate healing with strict instructions of rest. Gonzalo passed away in July 2020; however, I was fortunate to know him[25] and observe the richness of his knowledge and trust he amassed. I know he would be happy that I am sharing a particular incident which took place eight years ago.

A teenage boy was playing ball, and it escapes me now if it was soccer or basketball; however, he fell hard to the ground with his right leg in severe pain, rapidly swelling. His friends carried him to the home of the only Western health care provider in the village at that time. Juana Herrera, trained as an auxiliary nurse of the Panamanian Ministry of Health, delivered care for more than 30 years, was a trusted member of the community where she was born. Juana did everything from vaccinations to delivering babies, and she worked with very limited supplies and technology. No X-ray machines were available, and when necessary she would refer patients to larger island where there is a small hospital or to Panama City. In this situation she did neither. Once the family was informed, they called for the bone setter, Gonzalo. Juana stepped back to allow a change in diagnostician and prescribed therapy. The wide-eyed university students were aghast. First, they were alarmed that the community did not have an X-ray machine. Second, at a minimum, they felt the boy needed to get to the hospital. I politely pushed them back and quietly asked them to respect the decision and to observe and learn.

The parents had limited funds to send their child off the island. It would cost money for travel, stay, and food for at least one other family member that would have to accompany him. The university students wanted to chip in to offer help for medical care, while the family remained steadfast about not leaving the island. They respected their healer who worked on the teenager as he grimaced with increasing pain and swelling. Juana honored the family's decision since she understands the culture and the underlying factors that drive them to make such decisions.

While the students remained very concerned and would visit the boy at his home during homestays on the island, his leg remained restricted as did the healer's prescription for hammock rest. The Westernized college students worried about the teenage boy's long-term damage, while his Guna friends were more interested in when he'll be ready to play ball. Not surprising to me, I returned six months later to find the teenager playing with his friends, with no obvious damage. While this presents another anecdotal account, such examples offer insights into the role of history, culture, and this wider relationship to community health prevention, promotion, and treatment practices.

Conclusion

Population health is an intricate puzzle shaped by numerous disciplines, perspectives, stakeholders, and driven by who frames the issue. There are many competing health and health-related topics, priorities, and population challenges from community to national to regional and global levels. Issues range from local outbreaks to cross-border spread of food-, water-, and vector-borne diseases, rise in cancers, heart disease, strokes, diabetes, violence, mental health, and natural disasters and climate change causing displacement, disruption, and depression with old and new environmental health risks throughout the literature. With so many competing issues, we have to ask, where does a community start? Do they prioritize the deadliest community health threat, the best opportunity for success, the population most in need, the geographic location(s), the topic with the greatest political will and available funding, or another rationale for action? We may react to the fear of a serious disease, illness, or injury when it hits us close to home. We may travel or study abroad, watch a documentary, stream a YouTube clip, or know families, friends, or co-workers that experienced the horrific deadly disease, violent act, or devastation from a natural disaster. Our capricious responses signal the complexities of public health actions.

Notes

1 David Werner, *Donde No Hay Doctor* (*Where There Is No Doctor*) (Berkeley, CA: Hesperian Foundation, 1970). Now translated into over 100 languages; as of 2017 there have been 15 revised editions of this book.

2 Carlos Monge, Pan American Health Organization, *Sixteenth Meeting of the PAHO Advisory Committee on Medical Research* (July 11–15, 1977, Washington, DC).

3 World Health Organization and UNICEF, *Inequalities in Sanitation and Drinking Water in Latin America and the Caribbean* (Joint report), (Geneva and New York: WHO and UNICEF, 2016).

4 Amanda Glassman and Miriam Temin, eds. "Case 5: A Solid Foundation for Child Health – Mexico's *Piso Firme* Program," in *Millions Saved: New Cases of Proven Success in Global Health* (Washington, DC: Center for Global Development, 2016), 48–57.

5 Oxfam and Enough: Together We Can End Violence against Women, *Executive Summary: Breaking the Mould: The Changing Belief Systems and Gender Norms to Eliminate Violence against Women*, July 2008, https://oxfamilibrary.openrepository.com/bitstream/handle/10546/620524/rr-breaking-the-mould-250718-summ-en.pdf, and "High Rates of Violence against Women in Latin America Despite Femicide Legislation: Possible Steps Forward," *The Dialogue: Leadership for the Americas*, https://www.thedialogue.org/blogs/2018/10/high-rates-of-violence-against-women-in-latin-america-despite-femicide-legislation-possible-steps-forward/.

6 Horst W.J. Rittel and Melvin M. Webber, "Dilemmas in General Theory of Planning," *Policy Sciences* 4 (1973): 155–169.

7 Helen Walls, "Wicked Problems and 'Wicked' Solutions," *Globalization and Health* 14, no. 34 (2018). https://doi.org/10.1186/s12992-018-0353-x.

8 Marcos Cueto and Steven Palmer, *Medicine and Public Health in Latin America* (Cambridge: Cambridge University Press, 2015).

9 See *Public Health in England: The Report of the Committee of Inquiry into the Future Development of the Public Health Function* (London: HMSO, 1988) and the World Health Organization website, https://www.euro.who.int/en/health-topics/Health-systems/public-health-services/public-health-services.

10 R.C. Virchow, "Report on the Typhus Epidemic in Upper Silesia," *America Journal of Public Health* 96, no. 12 (December 2006): 2102–2105.

11 Howard Waitzkin et al., "Social Medicine Then and Now: Lessons from Latin America," *American Journal of Public Health* 91, no. 10 (October 2001): 1598.

12 Ibid, 1593.
13 Julie Feinsilver, *Healing the Masses* (Berkeley, CA: University of California Press, 1993).
14 David Werner, "Health Care in Cuba: A Model Service or a Means of Social Control – or Both?" in *Practicing Health for All*, eds. David Morley, Jon E. Rohde and Glen Williams (Oxford: Oxford University Press, 1983), 17–37.
15 Pedro Coutlin-Churchman, "The 'Cuban Epidemic Neuropathy' of the 1990s: A Glimpse from Inside a Totalitarian Disease," *Surgical Neurology International* 5, no. 84 (2014). https://surgicalneurologyint.com/surgicalint-articles/the-cuban-epidemic-neuropathy-of-the-1990s-a-glimpse-from-inside-a-totalitarian-disease/
16 Dr. Jason Harris, Associate Professor of Pediatrics at Harvard Medical School in an interview with *Drug Development & Discovery Magazine*, as quoted in Joanne Van Zuidam, "CDC Recommends Cholera Vaccine for U.S. Travelers," *R&D World*, May 19, 2017, https://www.rdworldonline.com/cdc-recommends-cholera-vaccine-for-u-s-travelers.
17 The World Health Organization on May 26, 2017, announced the awarding of the Dr. Lee Jong-wook Memorial Prize for Public Health to the Henry Reeve International Medical Brigade (Cuba). See http://www.who.int/mediacentre/events/2017/wha70/lee-jong-wook-prize/en/, accessed July 25, 2017.
18 Human Rights Watch, *World Report 2017*, accessed July 25, 2017, https://www.hrw.org/world-report/2017/country-chapters/cuba.
19 John R. Pierce and Jim Writer, *Yellow Jack: How Yellow Fever Ravaged America and Walter Reed Discovered Its Deadly Secrets* (Hoboken, NJ: J. Wiley, 2005), 77.
20 Ibid, 14.
21 "The South and Its Invader," *New York Tribune*, September 11, 1897, ProQuest Historical Newspapers: New York Tribune (1841–1922), 6.
22 Nichole Maxwell, *Witch-Doctor's Apprentice: Hunting for Medicinal Plants in the Amazon* (New York: Citadel Press, 1961).
23 Philip Bennett, "In Search of Native Medicine," *The Washington Post*, January 8, 1983, https://www.washingtonpost.com/archive/lifestyle/1983/01/08/in-search-of-native-medicine/08e1e6c1-44f4-4236-9656-ae0dd8697a4f/.
24 George M. Foster, "On the Origin of Humoral Medicine in Latin America," *Medical Anthropology Quarterly*, n.s., 1, no. 4 (December 1987): 355–393.
25 James Howe, noted anthropologist and professor emeritus from MIT, provides decades of research on Guna culture and history. Gonzalo referred to "Jim" and one of his sons. In Chapter 5 some of Howe's key works are listed in both the bibliography of selected books and in the endnotes.

Bibliography – Selected Books

Abel, Christopher. *Health, Hygiene and Sanitation in Latin America c1870–c.1950*. London: Institute of Latin American Studies, 1996.
Allende, Salvador Gossens. *La Realidad Médico-Social Chilena*. Santiago: Ministerio de Salubriadad, Previsión y Asistencia Social, 1939.
Beaglehole, Robert, ed. *Global Public Health: A New Era*. Great Britain: Oxford University Press, 2003.
Cueto, Marcos and Palmer, Steven. *Medicine and Public Health in Latin America: A History*. Cambridge: Cambridge University Press, 2015.
Fay, Marianne, Andres Luis, Alberto, Fox, Charles, Narloch, Ulf, and Slawson, Michael. *Rethinking Infrastructure in Latin America and the Caribbean: Spending More to Achieve Better*. Washington, DC: World Bank Publications. ProQuest Ebook Central, 2017.

Frenk, Julio and Hoffman, Steven J., eds. *"To Save Humanity," What Matters Most for a Healthy Future*. New York: Oxford University Press, 2015.

Foster, George M. *Hippocrates Latin American Legacy: Humoral Medicine in the New World*. New York: Routledge, 1994.

Maxwell, Nicole. *Witchdoctor's Apprentice – Hunting for Medicinal Plants in the Amazon*. New York: Citadel Press 3rd Edition, 1990.

McMichael, A.J. *Planetary Overload: Global Environmental Change and he Health of the Human Species*. Cambridge: Cambridge University Press, 1993.

Pan American Health Organization. *International Health: A North South Debate*. Washington, DC: PAHO, 1992.

Werner, David. *Where There Is No Doctor, Hesperian Foundation*. Berkley, MI: Hesperian Foundation, October 1977 (updated version May 1992).

2
DEVELOPMENT AND PUBLIC HEALTH

The great news is that health outcomes have improved with 98% of children in Latin America able to reach their first birthday as compared to only 75% one hundred years ago. The disturbing news is that while the life expectancy in Chile and Costa Rica is greater than 80 years, this is in contrast to Bolivia, Guyana, and Haiti where life expectancy is below 70 years. Haiti reported the lowest in the region with 64 years.[1] Statistics expose the inequality in human development, and the consequent challenges that exist both within and across countries in the region. Sadly, Latin America and the Caribbean remains the most unequal region in the world today.

There are stark realities of devastating public health outcomes where poverty prevails. The heart wrenching images of tiny babies with small heads in Recife, Brazil, weakened by the Zika virus, trigger a visceral reaction of sadness, tragedy, and fear all rolled into one. Yet our attention is often not drawn to the root causes of these conditions. We tend to focus on the problem rather than the issues that underlie these problems. This is what Sir Michael Marmot refers to as the causes of disease and the significance of the social and societal determinants of health. We want to ease the pain of the child while the mother coddles to comfort the crying sick babies. We too often react without focusing the attention on the complexity of the underlying issues. These are immense social problems that necessitate a broader understanding of the many interconnected factors necessary for the implementation of targeted policies and actions in response to human suffering.

Measuring Population Health and Development

Life expectancy is the simplest measure of health in a population. We know life expectancies can differ within and across countries based upon the underlying

DOI: 10.4324/9781003007401-3

social, economic, political, and environmental conditions taking into account gender identity, race, ethnicity, age, and location of where one lives and works. The practice of using a single health status indicator, such as infant mortality rate (IMR), to assess human health and development may only provide a snapshot view and avoid the deep dive analysis. IMR, a measure of infant deaths under the age of one, may be easier to capture than the under-five mortality rate (U5-MR); however, the U5-MR provides a more complete picture of the social and economic development index of where health is impacted within a population. The concept of using composite measures to evaluate public health and development has evolved over time. The use of the standard of living (gross national income), healthy life (life expectancy at birth) coupled with knowledge (literacy) rates helps quantify the potential for human development through economic, health, and education measures.

Human development is an important indicator of public health and identifies inequalities within and across nations. Since 1990 the United Nations Development Program has reported the Human Development Index (HDI), with measures available for 189 countries today. These composite indicators rank countries from very high, high, medium, and low levels of human development with a gradient measure, with 1.0 representing the highest score. The HDI report for Latin America and the Caribbean (2018) showed a very high development score for Chile ranking 44 (0.843), followed by Argentina 47 (0.825), Bahamas 54 (0.807), Uruguay 55 (0.804), and Barbados 58 (0.800). Conversely, Haiti ranked 168 (0.498) at the lowest human development level in the region, in contrast with Norway which ranked number 1 (0.953) in the world.[2]

The measure of inequalities within a country is not fully captured with the HDI since the averaging of aggregate data does not necessarily pinpoint such disparities. The Multidimensional Poverty Index (MPI), a collaboration of the UNDP and Oxford University's Poverty and Human Development Program, measures poverty beyond income and includes ten indicators. In 2019, the MPI revealed the wide variations within and across countries showing low- and middle-income countries with extensive subnational inequality of which children under 18 years of age suffer the greatest burden of multidimensional poverty. In Latin America, the MPI index and vulnerable population rates within countries are as follows: Guatemala has an MPI of 28.9 with 21.1% of the population vulnerable; Honduras has an MPI of 19.3 with 22.3% of the population vulnerable; and Bolivia has an MPI of 20.4 with 15.7% of the population vulnerable.[3]

While many Latin American and the Caribbean countries have made progress, there is no escaping the fact that the region continues to exhibit greater inequities. The 2019 Human Development Report for Latin America uncovers the intensity of population deprivation, which is an important dimension of poverty. Highest deprivation rates in Latin America are found in Bolivia (46%), Brazil (42.5%), Colombia (40.6%), Dominican Republic (38.9%) Ecuador (40%), El Salvador (41.2%), Guatemala (46.2%), Honduras (46.4%), and Mexico

(39.2%). Nobel Laureate of Economic Sciences (1998), Amartya Sen, introduced the relevancy of human capability as a driver to human development. In his book, *Development as Freedom*, he shows how the measures of deprivation and freedom are central to the public health and development process. Do we reduce population deaths through stimulating the economy for economic growth or do we invest in social well-being to reduce these deprivations? According to Sen, poverty is the deprivation of basic capacities and the lack of freedom that hinders development.[4] With such high rates of documented deprivation, the longer-term impact that COVID-19 will have on the region is a stark reminder of the vulnerabilities that require preventive interventions and policies to be more proactive to mitigate further decline.

Today, the Human Development Office includes other composite data reports beyond the HDI and MPI such as the Inequality-adjusted Human Development Index (IHDI), Gender Development Index (GDI), and Gender-Inequality index (GII). The IHDI combines achievements in a country for health, education, and income, but then assesses how this is distributed within a population using distribution-sensitive indices within each category. This is a more robust way to capture the distribution of inequalities of the HDI calculation. One limitation, however, is that it does not account for the overlapping inequalities. The data are useful for policies to improve human development by reducing inequality, if such strategies are actually implemented. This is especially important in the region due to greater gender inequalities.[5]

Women's health remains an important issue in Latin America and the Caribbean. For example, Argentina is predominately Roman Catholic with approximately 80% of the total population[6] and contraceptives were not available until 1985. Unsafe abortions account for more than 20% of maternal mortality in Latin America and 30% in Argentina.[7] While the maternal mortality rates have improved, disparities remain throughout the region. The availability, accessibility, and utilization of health and health-related service have improved. However, the rationale that such services are all available, although not utilized, needs further investigation into the overall inaccessibility related to financial, geographic, cultural, time, gender-associated barriers that thwart development.

According to the World Bank data (2015), 80% of the population in Latin America and 42% from the Caribbean small states reside in cities today. As presented in Chapter 1, the lack of a sound infrastructure remains a prevailing theme in public health, and where rural and indigenous populations continue to lack equal access to necessary services.

I have worked with marginalized populations in Latin America and the concern for reliable infrastructure and health development has not been achieved equally. Potable water systems may be threatened by design, spare parts, and bad weather, causing outbreaks of diarrheal disease as children drink untreated water and families struggle to find water for cooking and bathing. This often occurs because of a broken or unavailable PCV piping coupled with the political entanglements. However, the official data show potable water is available, while it is not consistently accessible. Safe water is necessary for life. It is arguably a universal human right, a social determinant of health, and yet not a reality for all. Nevertheless, it is evident that the availability and accessibility to cell phones today have reached faster and further into regions of the world than the realization of safe water, sanitation, and housing to meet population needs. In the 1980s, I asked the same question about how liters of Coca-Cola bottles reached the most remote areas and thought about the ingenuity of the marketing and distribution strategies of such multinational corporations in a globalizing world. Scrutinizing the role globalization plays in public health is instructive as it characterizes both the benefits and detriments to population health and will be covered in a subsequent chapter.

Inequalities and Development Approaches

Embracing public health issues as social problems is not simple to tackle. It requires a focus on prevention, with multiple strategies to get to the underlying root causes. This is where important contributions on inequalities in the region have been made by social scientists concerned with the social, cultural, economic, and political determinants of underdevelopment within and across countries throughout Latin America since post-World War II. It was German sociologist Max Weber in the late 19th century and early 20th century who proposed the theory of modernization, encouraging countries to move toward industrialization and embrace Westernized democratic values as the best path to development. This was advanced by economist William Rostow who provided the five stages to achieve economic development. Modernization theorists proposed that removing the economic, social, and cultural barriers would bring about a shift from underdevelopment to development. Refuting the modernization theory, scholars such as Raúl Prebish, Andre Gunder Frank, Fernando Cardoso, and Enrique Faletto proposed a different approach based upon the dependency theory. In the 1960s, dependency theorist in Latin America argued that it is the social and economic forces and class structures that are responsible for such global inequalities that shape imbalances in development within and across nations. Scholars maintained that underdevelopment in Latin America was a direct outcome of capital flows better understood within the historical and structural context of underdevelopment. Sociologist Immanuel Wallerstein expanded upon the dependency theory with the world systems perspective, further contending that the global economic system brought about social changes that ultimately benefit some countries while leaving others behind. Consequently, how a nation is integrated into such a global economic system will influence a country's level of economic development. Wallerstein divided the world system into core, periphery, and semi-periphery countries, and argues that it is the powerful core countries that dominant the periphery low-income countries and semi-periphry middle-income countries. His theory highlights the historical and social structure of inequality within the world economic system.[8] This is where multinational corporations and the commercial determinants of public health will be explored in Chapter 3. Development theories in Latin America certainly deserve much more attention than this book can offer. But what is important to recognize is that Latin American scholars have provided valuable contributions to understanding such structural determinants, the underlying social, cultural, economic, and political factors, which have been shown to have greater impacts on inequalities and health disparities.

The 1980s new neoliberal order in Latin America focused on social, economic, and political development. During this time, Latin American countries such as Brazil, Bolivia, Ecuador, El Salvador, and Venezuela were demanding health reforms to make health a right for all. This gained traction throughout Latin America. *Buen Vivir* (To Live Well) was introduced as a new path to development, critical for the existing focus on economic growth and increased consumption.[9] Development approaches throughout Latin America have had both direct and indirect impacts on population health. The 1940s Green Revolution arrived in Mexico in 1950s–1960s and spread throughout the Americas as well as the Alliance for Progress in 1961; they stand out as two important indirect population health considerations. It is also the 1970s–1980s oil shocks, the 1980s debt crisis, rise of neoliberal economic policies, and the 1990s International Monetary Fund's (IMF) Structural Adjustment Programs (SAPs) that had serious impacts on public health in Latin America during the 20th century. The IMF programs exacerbated the problems, when austerity measures required cutbacks to health and education programs.

Poverty and Beyond

The history of health in Latin America and the Caribbean extends beyond the measure of economic growth, even though this continues to dominate discussions about public health and development. The vicious cycle that perpetuated poverty and ill health is multidimensional. This requires a better appreciation of the human face of poverty where individuals may feel exploited and humiliated, powerless, and hopeless, with barriers to plan ahead for a better future, and sadly, to feel invisible.

Using a multidimensional perspective of poverty provides a more human face to the numerical value, and which poor health can be observed and measured. In a 1990s unprecedented World Bank project to document *The Voices of the Poor*, 60,000 people from 60 countries participated in sharing their personal perspectives on poverty. In the final report, *Voices of the Poor from Many Lands*, participatory research presented the testimonials of determination and resiliency of the poor across 14 countries, including Argentina, Brazil, Ecuador, and Jamaica in Latin America and the Caribbean.[10]

This research revealed common themes across countries. Similar concerns were associated with violence, crime, underemployment and unemployment, discrimination, inequality, lack of accessibility to services, contributing to the vicious cycle of poverty and poor health outcomes. A child in Ecuador need not shine shoes to pay for school expenses. The difficult decision to take off work and forfeit income so one can go to a health clinic is exacerbated by the cost of transportation and medicines, and cultural barriers of accessibility to services. Robert Chambers used the term "rachet effect" to further illustrate the existence of the vicious cycle of poor health and poverty.[11] This concept is further aggravated when a sick member of the family, especially a wage earner, falls ill and it becomes necessary to use any funds or borrow money. This will place the family into debt and increase impoverishment. The prevention of disease, disability, and death is linked to reducing situations of poverty and ultimately a path toward development. An unhealthy population is a less productive one; therefore, investing in health is both the ends and the means to development.

The World Bank estimated that 130 million people in Latin America and the Caribbean are chronically poor and confront many diseases due to extreme poverty, also referred to as neglected tropical diseases. Approximately 25 million people in the region are at high risk for malaria with 75% of the cases found alone in Brazil, Colombia, and Venezuela. This is the public health paradox. Some of the richest countries in the region like Argentina, Brazil, and Mexico are the ones that face high rates of poverty and high rates of diseases such as Chagas, schistosomiasis, malaria, and helminths.[12] A majority of American trypanosomiasis, also known as Chagas disease, is reported from Latin America where it is endemic in 21 countries with 8 million people infected.[13] It is transmitted by the reduviid bug that comfortably resides in crevices of poorly constructed homes and deposits infective feces into the skin when biting its human victim during nighttime activity. Argentina ranks very high on the HDI, placed at 47th out of 189 countries; however, it has one of the highest rates of Chagas. In Mexico, pregnant mothers transmit the disease to their newborns among the poorest population, and Brazil's 25% of the poorest population are living with Chagas. A regional example of Chagas disease and health diplomacy will be discussed further in Chapter 5.

Inequality Thwarts Development and Public Health

There has been much research and discussion on social inequalities in health for decades; yet, few countries have used the research to devise comprehensive plans for social and economic policies to respond to the blatant social ills that impact poor health outcomes. The World Health Organization's (WHO) Commission on Social Determinants of Health (CSDH) report (2008) made a compelling argument about why all sectors of the government are necessary to address public health policies for a more comprehensive response to tackle the social, cultural, economic, environmental, and political origins of poor health. Dr. Margaret Chan, former director general of the WHO, reminds us that the "[g]aps in health outcomes are not a matter of fate- they are indicators of policy failure."[14] This has not been easy since conflating the SDoH and social processes that shape such determinants with unequal distribution of resource can mislead policy.[15] Many were eager to embrace the WHO Commission's report. However, Vicente Navarro, while supporting the rigorous research conducted for this report, argued that the greatest weakness was in the wording, "social inequalities kills." Vincente disputed that "[i]t is not inequalities that kill, but those how benefit from the inequalities that kill."[16] Social equity is a rational way to practice public health, according to Carissa Etienne, PAHO Director. Inequities have become the structural threat to health and development. To do this she suggests better stewardship of the health sector to promote equity.[17] Unmistakably, this demands more than a health sector's involvement and must also consider income inequalities and related policies.

The Gini coefficient measures the distribution of income in a country from 0 to 1 with 0 reaching equality or 0% to 1 or 100% inequality. According to the Gini coefficient rankings, Brazil, Colombia, and Panama document unequal reporting of 51.3, 50.8 and 50.4, respectively, with Brazil at the highest income inequality in Latin America. A 2018 United Nations report revealed that poverty showed some decline in 2017, after rising in 2015 and 2016, while extreme poverty remained the same. This offers important insights into the demographic urban and rural disparities in the region.[18] Inequality reveals the socially determined differences in health status outcomes within and across countries and a weak public health sector will intensify the health inequities. Therefore, upgrading an integrated system to include equity-oriented social policies will improve public health outcomes. It is such political and society equity-oriented policies to improve the access to education, primary health care services, and nutrition that show the best results to strengthen human capital in Latin America and the Caribbean.

This has been done through direct cash transfers to households with specified conditions. One of the most rigorously researched evidence-based social development programs was launched in Mexico in 1997 under President Ernesto Zedillo. This conditional cash transfer (CCT) program used a multidimensional approach to tackle poverty through improving health, nutrition, and educational outcomes. Originally called *Progresa* (Progress) then *Oportunidades* (Opportunities), *Prospera* (Prosper), this program gave cash directly to families with the condition that they keep children in school, get health checkups, and attend nutritional training. Mexico, facing the challenge of keeping older girls in school, motivated families with increased sums to ensure girls would continue their education. While cash transfer programs began in Mexico, they spread throughout the region and have been adapted in more than 50 countries. The conditional component of cash transfers was argued as too paternalistic since families would only receive the funds if they agreed to specified conditions.

The removal of conditionality focused on result-based outcomes. Brazil's *Bolsa Familia*, initiated by President Luiz Ignacio "Lula" da Silva in 2003, is the largest cash transfer program in the world today. While there were earlier social protection initiatives in Latin America before the inception of Mexico's *Progresa's* program, such *as Programa de Asignación Familiar* (Program of Family Assignment) in Honduras supported through the Inter-American Development Bank (IDB) and Brazil's zero hunger effort, it was Mexico's rigorous approach to integrate CCT for health, education, and nutrition that makes it the first.

The Global Financing Facility (GFF) of the World Bank is a newer strategy for international development financing, including two countries in Latin America and the Caribbean, i.e. Guatemala and Haiti. The GFF model bridges the leadership and investments of governments in which the programs will be implemented, in coordination with international donors, and private sectors such as foundations or businesses. In November 2018, $1 billion dollar was pledged from world leaders to support a multi-stakeholder partnership targeting efforts to improve the health of women, children, and adolescents. Based upon Smart Financing for Evidence-based interventions, Scaled Financing will mobilize other funds, and reflect Sustainable Financing. A good example is *Crecer Sano* (Growing Healthy), a Guatemala Nutrition and Health Project from 2016 to 2020. This project was in response to Guatemala reporting the highest rates of malnutrition (46.5%) in Latin America and the Caribbean, with higher rates (61%) among indigenous populations.[19] The underlying factors to address include chronic malnutrition, lack of access to safe water and sanitation, poor maternal health, poor child feeding practices, and adequate health services, with less than 50% of the population having access to regular primary health care services.[20]

Once again, it brings us to the discussion of establishing a public health infrastructure beyond the health sector. *Crecer Sano* is a broad partnership between Guatemala and the Governments of Canada, Norway, World Bank, and the Bill and Melinda Gates Foundation with a funding commitment of $100 million to combat malnutrition in pregnant women, children under two years of age with high rates of chronic malnutrition, and a specific target on the vulnerable indigenous population. The strategy was to combine health and education in response to severe malnutrition. Guatemala's Minister of Finance Julio Héctor Estrada remarked how the loan would be helpful in…

> reducing malnutrition we will increase the productivity of our future work force. We are also thankful for the grant from the GFF which will allow us to benefit from better loan terms and thereby channel more resources to vulnerable populations in Guatemala.[21]

A renewed GFF initiative is underway by the Guatemalan Government for 2020–2024, *Cruzada Nacional por la Nutrición* (A Crusade for Better Nutrition), with the promise to improve education, health, and nutrition. This includes multisector participation of social development, economic and finance, communication and infrastructure, education, agriculture, farming and food, international cooperation, government departments of health in municipalities, local governments, private sector, civil society, and a robust monitoring and evaluation component.[22]

While extreme poverty declined and middle class showed robust growth in Latin America and the Caribbean, the most impoverished became invisible and left behind. Research has shown that the more equalitarian a political, economic, and social system is, the less health inequalities will exist. The 1980s revealed that good health at low cost could be achieved when governments made the political and social commitment to meet the basic needs for all, provide equal access to health and education for both boys and girls with equitable distribution across urban and rural populations, and monitor sufficient nutritional intake.

1980s Debt Crisis Collides with Public Health

For many countries in Latin America, the 1980s will be remembered as a period of escalating poverty and malnutrition and plummeting of health indicators. UNICEF documented Latin American countries' deteriorating health situation with evidence of increasing incidence of infectious diseases such as typhoid, gastrointestinal diseases, hepatitis, tuberculosis, malaria, and yaws.[23] Chile's commitment to protect the high-risk populations through providing health care, education, nutritional surveillance, and subsidies for the most vulnerable population showed success in the early 1980s. However, in 1986, a PAHO report revealed that Chile's targeted interventions were no longer meeting the needs. Even Costa Rica, which documented impressive health outcomes with a low-cost equity-oriented approach and urban and rural investments in both health and education, showed stagnating infant and child mortality rates.[24] Good health at low-cost research showed that Costa Rica in the Western Hemisphere and China, Kerala (India), and Sri Lanka were able to achieve significant health improvements by implementing intersectoral policies, which included the SDoH well beyond the narrow focus of health systems. This included the specific commitment to equitable approaches to meet human basic needs, education for all, urban rural equitable distribution of social services, monitoring food intake in sufficient quantities, and the political will to ensure that all the above-mentioned points were met. Clearly, different approaches across different political systems in countries were implemented. Costa Rica confronted great economic challenges during the debt crisis with strict austerity measures put into place by the World Bank and IMF. The IMR in Brazil increased by 12% in 1984. In fact by 1982, the IMR jumped from 65 deaths per 1,000 to 73 per 1,000.[25] Economist presented two major factors contributed to the deteriorating economic conditions in Latin American nations, i.e. the external debt crisis and the drastically reduced levels of foreign capital.

The debts were largely the result of fluctuating oil prices in 1973 and 1979 coupled with increasing borrowing as oil-producing countries turned their surplus into loans. Anticipating that oil prices would remain high in combination with low interest rates, even the oil exporting nations of Latin America, Mexico and Venezuela, borrowed heavily in the 1970s. Argentina and Brazil with thriving economies before the debt crisis also borrowed heavily to build their infrastructure. While there was some good news of economic growth, the bad news was the accumulation of massive debt at variable interest rates. As a result, the combination of recession and high interest rates in the United States and other rich nations raised the cost of servicing the debt while reducing imports from poorer countries. This, in turn, reduced both the amount and costs of primary exports by debtor countries, bringing about the crisis. The renegotiation of existing debt was made contingent on an agreement between the IMF and debtor nations. Most of the Latin American countries were forced to enter into such agreements to reduce deficits and control their inflation in exchange for receiving emergency loans. As the crisis loomed, the ability to repay debt, and even to service the interest rates, became impossible. While it was Mexico's finance minister in 1982 who first called for a moratorium on debt repayment with their inability to meet repayment deadlines, this ultimately brought about a refusal of the financial institutions to provide any loans to Latin America. Subsequently, countries agreed to the IMF's austerity programs with direct and indirect impacts on population health.[26] This brief overview of the 1980s debt crisis in Latin America is important to understand how the external economic conditions had a serious impact on health status and access to health services as national economies adjusted internally.

The IMF was never designed to lend money to developing countries, nor to promote the development or redistribution of wealth; rather, it functions as a short-term fix. In fact, the IMF did not contain any methods to protect the neediest members of the society against austerity measures.[27] Yet when Latin American countries turned to the IMF, their balance of payment problems and severe austerity measures caused a major reduction in expenditures on health and education. On the other hand, the World Bank focused on longer-term development strategies. The demand for a better approach to the human reality of development became fully realized during this debt crisis since the austerity measures and structural adjustment disproportionately impacted sub-Saharan African and Latin American countries. The World Bank and the IMF influenced all economic policies at this time. The UNICEF was the first international organization to identify the negative impacts such policies were having on populations, with evidence showing worsening child malnutrition and deteriorating health of women and children in the poorest populations, and they brought in other key stakeholders to address the negative impacts on health, education, and nutrition of children.[28] The case studies from Latin America exposed something not previously identified, i.e. the disproportionate impact the debt crisis had on women.[29]

Public versus Private Good Controversy for Public Health

In order for public health to be a public good it needs to be both nonexclusionary and nonrivalrous. For example, the air we breathe shows everyone has equal access to air and breathing air does not restrict another person's availability to this same air. There are both negative and positive externalities of a public good to understand the public health impact. One may do everything possible to keep their air clean, by reducing carbon emission and minimizing pollutions, and still they may be forced to breathe poor quality air causing lung, heart, or eye-related health issues within a population. This is the negative externalities of such a public good. The positive side is that you may be a major polluter and still benefit from better air to breathe since others are doing their job to protect the air. This has been seen in the growing megacities in Latin America, Mexico City, and Rio de Janeiro faced with growing threats of air quality due to industrial development, urbanization, and population growth.

Today we observe the positive externalities of another public good, that is vaccines. Vaccinations in Latin America has increased throughout the 20th and 21st centuries, allowing the population to achieve "herd immunity." Herd immunity is when the threshold to protect a population is achieved, even if everyone has not been exposed to the germ or vaccinated. This is important as recent measles outbreak increased in the Americas, with the Argentine Ministry of Health reporting almost 100 cases in 2019, and more than 120 cases of chickenpox in Chihuahua, Mexico in a migrant camp, according to the Ministry of Labor and Social Welfare. This is totally preventable with vaccinations.

Why the reemergence of measles? While there is more than one simplistic answer, in part, the increase in vaccine hesitancy and the rise in anti-vaxxer social movements have left more people at risk. When populations refuse vaccination for religious, lifestyle, or other rationales, herd immunity may not be met and the spread will threaten unprotected and susceptible populations, including the very young, old, immunocompromised populations and those receiving chemotherapy or living with HIV/AIDS. This is especially relevant for measles since it requires 90–95% of the population to be vaccinated in order to reach herd immunity. It is no surprise with increased globalization, population shifts, and displacement that this is becoming more of a challenge to prevent and protect populations.

Historically it was a challenge to get vaccines to rural communities or health centers with poor roads, limited access, or during rainy seasons when roads become impassable. The cold chain provided a temperature-controlled system used to ensure the storage, transport, and distribution of vaccines from manufacture to the point of use is maintained even when confronted with potential logistical and management barriers. Both chickenpox (varicella) and the combined measles, mumps, and rubella (MMR) vaccines require such care. During the 1980s, I remember seeing boxes of vaccines sitting in the direct sun or on small runways in Central and South American airports due to an unexpected delay in retrieving them. Keeping vaccines at the right temperature was also a challenge. Vaccines were sometimes placed in small refrigerators where inconsistent electricity or regulating cooling temperatures were also used to chill beverages, meats, and other food requiring refrigeration. It was a good thing that new vaccine refrigerator technology came along with easy-to-read temperature controls, slots specific to storing vaccines, and back-up propane during intermittent blackouts or when no electricity was available. The cold chain made a great contribution to reducing child diseases throughout Latin America and the Caribbean.

The question of public health as public good continues to conflict with a private good analysis from the access and purchase of safe water. The 1980s opened the door to two approaches to health care. The first approach was market driven and reached populations that were insured through private institutions and required social security as well as access to private health care services, while the second approach was a public health system to reach the poor and those without insurance, requiring public health care services. The first, a more robust system, exemplified the commodification of health and eventually embraced the privatization of health from the financing, managing to the delivery of service in the 1990s. Private health care institutions dominated health care services during the health sector reform period that began in the 1990s.[30]

From Primary Health Care (1978) to Millennium Development Goals (2000–2015) to Sustainable Development Goals (2015–2030)

Since the 1970s the notion of collective health has been integrated into the wider economic and social development discourse in Latin America. The idea that illnesses and diseases were related to social conditions gave rise to social medicine in Latin America. Social movements created new efforts for social medicine and more awareness about the underlying determinants that contributed to poor health outcomes. However, where individual countries took actions to tackle prevailing issues of poverty, unemployment, lack of sanitation and hygiene, poor nutrition, and substandard housing, the political will to respond remained uneven within and across countries. The trajectory of change, over a span of more than four decades, can be observed through three ambitious strategies.

Possibly, it was the 1978 landmark international health conference in Alma-Ata, Russia (today known as Almaty, Kazakhstan) to seek Health for All by the Year 2000 (HFA2000) that provided the foundation for both public health and development and health security. The Health for All philosophy proposed a commitment of health resources, with the allocation of such resources rooted in the fundamental principles of equity, community participation, and collaboration through intersectoral approaches within and across countries. This occurred during the Cold War, which may explain why, in part, the United States did not participate in this first international health conference whereby Health for All was proposed as a commitment to social justice with accessible equitable resource allocation. Within the HFA2000 doctrine, primary health care is seen as the essential health care that is practical, scientifically sound, social and culturally acceptable, technologically accessible, incorporated into a health system, with central function and, equally important, integrated into the social and economic strategies of a nation.

> Primary care is essential health care based on practical, scientifically sound and socially acceptable methods and technology made universally accessible to individuals and families in the community through their full participation and at a cost that the community and country can afford in the spirit of self-reliance and determination.[31]

It has its roots in three principles: equity, community participation, and collaboration across many sectors, extending beyond the medical and health fields. Primary health care sought to reduce health inequalities by including the social and economic sectors and political characteristics of a country more seamlessly, while engaging community participation. To achieve this, health systems would need to restructure, prioritize the primary levels of care, and ensure social justice and equitable distribution of resources were met. Costa Rica's commitment began with disbanding a permanent military and reallocate funds to improve health, education, and the social contract to protect its citizens. This dramatic shift was actually initiated in 1948 in a joint effort between the Defense Minister and President José Figueres to call for a change to the constitution. This proposal presented an argument for assembling a civilian police force in place of permanent military force.

While the Primary Health Care/Health for All by 2000 initiative was not achieved, the United Nations (UN) put forth the Millennium Development Goals (MDGs) 2000–2015. The MDGs proposed eight targets for human development, of which three were directly related to health and the other five represented indirect impacts. Goal 4 was to improve child health, Goal 5 was to improve maternal health, and Goal 6 was to reduce infectious diseases such as HIV/AIDS, malaria, and tuberculosis (Table 2.1). Clearly, this was a broad approach; nevertheless, it showed the global commitment to public health and development. In 2008, 30 years after Alma-Ata, the Secretary General of the WHO, Margaret Chan, pronounced that "The Millennium Declaration and its Goals breathed new life into the values of equity and social justice, this time with a view toward ensuring the benefits of globalization are more evenly distributed between countries"[32].

The shift to the United Nations Sustainable Development Goals (SDGs) of 2015–2030 became a holistic approach to identify the direct and indirect impact of development to include the five Ps: People, planet, prosperity, peace,

TABLE 2.1 United Nations Millennium Development Goals (2000–2015)

Goals	Targets
Goal 1	Eradicate extreme poverty and hunger
Goal 2	Seek universal primary education
Goal 3	Promote gender equality and empowerment of women
Goal 4	Improve child health
Goal 5	Improve maternal mortality
Goal 6	Reduce infectious diseases (HIV/AIDS, malaria, tuberculosis, and other diseases)
Goal 7	Promote environmental sustainability
Goal 8	Develop global partnerships

Source: United Nations Millennium Development Goals (MDGs). No targets were developed for noncommunicable diseases or public health issues associated with globalization.

TABLE 2.2 United Nations Sustainable Development Goals (2015–2030)

Goals	Targets
Goal 1	No poverty
Goal 2	Zero hunger
Goal 3	Good health and well-being
Goal 4	Quality education
Goal 5	Gender equality
Goal 6	Clean water and sanitation
Goal 7	Affordable and clean energy
Goal 8	Decent work & economic growth
Goal 9	Industrial innovation and infrastructure
Goal 10	Reduced inequalities
Goal 11	Sustainable cities and communities
Goal 12	Responsible consumption and production
Goal 13	Climate action
Goal 14	Life below water
Goal 15	Life on land
Goal 16	Peace justice and institutions
Goal 17	Partnerships for the goal

Source: United Nations Sustainable Development Goals (2015–2030).

and partnerships. It focuses on achieving peace, prosperity, and well-being of people and the planet coupled with development of natural systems, and leadership through partnerships for better governance. It is not a linear process and requires broader acceptance of development challenges and realities. Consequently, without the adherence to the transdisciplinary study, research, and implementation of policies, the reality of achieving sustainable health development will never be fully realized (Table 2.2).

Case Study 2.1

Reflections from the Field: **Cristo Viajero** *Bogotá, Colombia*

As an idealistic Peace Corps Volunteer growing up in Long Island, New York and later living in Miami, Florida, I never experienced dire poverty upfront and close until I arrived in Bogotá, Colombia during the late 1970s. Sure, I read about abject poverty during the French Revolution in Charles Dickinson's *A Tale of Two Cities, Paris and London* (1775–1792), where he shows the destitution and misery of lower class, and the social ills of society's widespread hunger and malnutrition. I saw the graphic and disturbing newspaper pictures of people living on less than $1 per day, but my perspective changed in an instant the day I was abruptly stopped on a street in downtown Bogotá. *Que desea un bebe? ¡Ayúdeme!* (Do you want a baby? Help me!) With minimal Spanish proficiency at this time, I kept walking, as did the desperate girl following along with her crying newborn baby. I wondered, what could possibly drive someone to beg a stranger to take her baby? Bogotá was quickly emerging as one of the most violent cities in the world with a shamefully growing problem of street children – derogatorily termed *gamines* (street urchins). I thought of the sad human faces behind this disturbing moniker; yet I found many girls among the street children, contrary to the assumption that they were all dirty young boys living in sewers or in alley ways. I was moved by the young girls with their empty and desperate stares. This left an indelible impression that even 42 years later is memorable.

Cristo Viajero

It was an American priest and Colombian nun who became the pioneers helping the young girls and women with a program called *Cristo Viajero* (Wandering Christ). The American priest, *Padre Carlos Frijole* (Father Charles Bean), an extraordinary man of the cloth standing 6'6" and 300 pounds, invited me to work with them while I continued my language and cultural training. As it turned out, I would be able to continue my Peace Corps service working with the group on such an exciting innovative program to help disenfranchised women who work as low-paid sex workers in Bogotá, Colombia. It was the nun, *Hermana* (Sister) Angela Betancourt, who provided the cultural and spiritual connection for this endeavor. It did not matter to her that the young women were trying to survive as low-paid sex workers. And it did not seem to matter that *Cristo Viajero's* home base was a musty, cold, and dreary rundown building housed between ruins in a section of the center city known as *El Parque Voto Nacional*. There you could find Colombia's version of the FBI, *Departamento Administrativo de Seguridad* (DAS), with their offices close by, as were the local police.

I was intimidated by thugs and pimps who felt my work with these poorly compensated girls and women would cut into their unjust profits. Peace Corps insisted that I relocate to a safer job. After unyielding pleas and support from Sister Angela and Father Bean, a compromise was reached. I could stay as long as I agreed to have an escort in and out of the area.

My most dedicated escort was Olga. She was adequately equipped with a 10-inch knife that she carried deep inside her undergarments and kept close to her body. She was older than others and she was both experienced and respected on the streets. Olga did her best to care for her four children with the youngest, Jenny, just three years old. She wanted her kids to have better opportunities for education and a job that would provide food, housing, and a way to make them feel safe and secure. What mother wouldn't? This is a universal sentiment that I found throughout the world and is fundamental to understanding just how far a mother would go to provide for her children. The role of women in the *machismo* society of the 1970s paints a different picture than one today, notwithstanding the gender inequities and gender-based violence. Olga became my friend and my confidante as she struggled to balance her work, life, and care for her children. The face of poverty is seen through the eyes of this dedicated and hardworking woman.

I initially arrived to work on health education projects for these women such as nutrition, hygiene, and prevention against sexually transmitted infections at a time before the arrival of the HIV/AIDS pandemic. Clearly, however, the problems were much deeper. I soon learned that the girls as young as 13 years of age, some pregnant, were sniffing glue and popping pills as their only solace to minimize their perpetual pain. Many of these girls arrived from rural communities, *campesinos* (peasants), and were invisible in the capital city of Bogotá. They fled their homes without any formal education or skills. The city offered an escape from the physical and mental torment in their isolated homes. Consequently, the streets provided a strange safe haven where they could pilfer supplies or sell sexual services to earn money for food, goods, and, on their own terms, experience less pain. The indominable spirit and their survival was both sad, and, yes, impressive.

The program, *Cristo Viajero*, was a new endeavor. It began as a meeting space for both spiritual and personal guidance, as well as a hot meal. I tried to introduce the benefit of eating and cooking with vegetables, which not surprisingly, the women immediately rejected as irrelevant. They opined that such food sources were better used as animal feed. My unwelcomed health education program was my early introduction to why it is important to know your population, include recipients of any program development, and never seek to adopt a well-conceived program from one place to another. Strategies will always need to be adapted to meet the needs of the local population. Equally important, it taught me that it is never a helpful practice to tell someone what is best for them, without fully respecting the cultural relevancy.

During my stay the women were taught to make brooms and mops so they could sell the finished goods to local store owners. While all shopkeepers needed a broom, it was the motivation of *Hermana* Angela to give these girls and women the training, self-confidence, and dignity to succeed. I observed why self-esteem is an important characteristic to break the cycle of poverty. The development of a cottage industry grew from donations of sewing and silk-screening machines to contracts with local shopkeepers. *Hermana* Angela taught me how coupling health promotion with educational and spiritual guidance, with skill-based training could provide an economic alternative for these women and young girls. Further, it provided the freedom to be self-sufficient, gain confidence, hope, and a new path toward providing better nutrition and housing, and access to health services for their children.

The Story Continues

The story of Olga and her family does not end there. The tragedy is Olga was killed on the same streets she knew so well, and where I first met her. It was a violent time in Colombia. The U.S. Ambassador, Diego Asencio (1977–1980), was kidnapped by Colombia's paramilitary terrorist group known as *Alianza Democrática M-19* (April 19th Movement). On February 27, 1980 Ambassador Asencio was snatched during an afternoon event at the Dominican Republic's Embassy, while celebrating their Independence Day. After two months in captivity, he along with 16 other hostages, of which 12 were other Ambassadors, flew to Havana, Cuba as demanded by their captors. While in captivity the Red Cross provided the necessary aid for both hostages and captors, and Father Bean shared with me his participation behind the scenes. The political dimension of the paramilitary threat, prior to the rise of the drug cartel, highlights the impact of the dimensions of development in Colombia, where violence and health cannot be excluded. Admittedly, I was naïve and would say that health was separate from politics.

My naivety vanished, seized by the stark reality that public health, poverty, and politics, in Latin America and throughout the globe, remain inextricably linked.

I wish Olga knew the great impact she had on me. More importantly, I wish she knew her youngest children were safe. Father Bean, in coordination with the U.S. Embassy, helped an American family adopt her two younger children. I know through the many Sunday picnics I shared with Olga and her children she would be smiling. Her cherished children achieved everything she had hoped for, which is the access to high-quality education, good health, and a better way of life away from crime, violence, and poverty. I learned this is a universal wish of all mothers.

Conclusion

It is remarkable that as a 20-something-year-old volunteer, I was able to see the spectrum of struggles for many urban single women in Latin America, from the anguish of a terrified young teenage mother pleading with me to take her crying baby, to Olga's unwavering commitment to educate both me and her children about life challenges, to the empty sad stares of young destitute girls that would turn into smiles and hugs with the small investments of giving them the tools and skills to have a healthy and safe life.

This is what Amartya Sen would call support led investments in development, investing in people and giving them the tools, the freedom to succeed. I would say President John F. Kennedy knew exactly what he was doing in creating Peace Corps in 1961. I embraced the third objective of Peace Corps to educate others about the situations abroad. I continued to work with *Cristo Viajero*, after leaving Colombia due to the escalating violence, by writing small grants during the 1980s. I visited often, as I passed through on my way to the banks of the Magdalena River, working on tropical disease field research in collaboration with the Colombia Army, which will be presented later in the chapter on security and public health.

Four decades later, the interconnectedness of health, poverty, and development remains problematic. We know the issues. We acknowledge the underlying factors. We continue to depend upon the political will to invest in all people equally, in order to break the vicious cycle of poverty, violence, and poor health outcomes. Olga's reckoning that a mother would do anything it takes to keep her children healthy and safe is as apropos today as it was then.

Reflections from the Field: Women and Economic Development

I am thankful for the best hands-on educational opportunities I received. These were the lessons I learnt in the field, delivered not by experts but by the many brave, hardworking, and caring women, mothers, and grandmothers. These earlier experiences provide me with a greater appreciation of the fortitude of women throughout Latin America and the Caribbean. Nevertheless, even with decades of experience, there is always a reminder that we cannot neglect the daily struggles of a poor mother juggling far too many competing demands.

I was humbled by an experience in 2007, in a small community in the Ica Valley in Peru located 48 kilometers from the capital city of Lima. More importantly, I was embarrassed after 28 years of field work. I was invited by a colleague to collaborate on development projects with communities still trying to rebuild after the El Niño related *huayco* (mudslides) in 1998. Shortly after the small community-driven projects began a 7.9 earthquake struck devastated these same communities in the Ica Valley. This will be discussed further in Chapter 4 on disasters and climate crisis, but it is apropos to share an important lesson about the role of women, poverty, and economic development.

One community development project was to raise and sell *cuy* (guinea pigs) since the residents said they learned to monetize the export of these animals. Even though I might not have welcomed such a project, I respected the community's decision to do what they felt familiar and in their own best interest. The funds were raised to provide modules for guinea pig breeding by local families. The decision to raise the animals on a large landowner's property was agreed upon by all 23 families in this small community. It is important to recognize that Ica is an agricultural mecca and major agro-export business are cotton, asparagus, grapes, artichokes, along with 50 different products for export worldwide, all of which generates income for more than a half-million workers in the region. The agreement for families to rotate a feeding and care schedule for their shared guinea pig project ultimately fell upon the women even though the men established this arrangement. During one of my site visits I came upon guinea pigs without food or water mid-day and asked the project representative what happened. We scanned the schedule, identified the family responsible for that day, and we went to their home. Upon arrival a frenzied woman carrying one baby and holding the hand of a toddler came running out of the house. She apologized saying she could not travel to the site because she did not have any transportation and her husband went off to work. This was further complicated by the fact that on this same day it was her turn to cook for the community feeding program. All this was placed on this young woman without anyone recognizing that she was required to do double duty on the same day. She had no transport, no home or cellular phone to communicate, and no support. I was disheartened. Once again, I was reminded about the perpetual struggles of women. She only wanted to show me the milled alfalfa and water ready to feed the guinea pigs, which was soon delivered. This gave me the opportunity to talk to her and learn another important lesson about the perception of ownership. In placing the guinea pigs on the landowner's property, and not their own land, the feeling of ownership offered a different perspective from the poor working family where many are employed by the property owner. While they understood this was a project to help families, and all parties decided upon its location, the women were left with the added burden. Furthermore, they did not have the same sentiment given that animals were not physically situated on their own property. I should have known better. In post-disaster phases vulnerable communities will always disproportionately impact women. We are never too old to learn lessons and embrace our humility.

Case Study 2.2

Reflections from the Field – Ashley's First International Field Experience

It is often said that the memories of a first international experience will remain with you forever. It did for me. However, I also know that first impressions will not provide a complete understanding of a situation. This prompts further inquiry. I've seen this with the many university students I've taken abroad for the first time. I also saw this in 1995 when I took my seven-year-old daughter, Ashley, to visit *Cristo Viajero* (Case Study 2.1). This was my first international field experience, and I wanted to share this with her.

Here we were, 16 years later, observing a slightly more established program, and yet, the dimensions of poverty, with the indirect and direct impact on the health of the women and young girls, remained sadly familiar to me. Albeit now, I had a much greater depth of understanding the complexities of the issues. I also knew Ashley had already formed a very different picture in her seven-year-old mind about what poverty looked like. This was shaped by her first experience, her first impression, while visiting an indigenous community in Guna Yala, Panama.

Background

In 1991 I traveled to Guna Yala, Panama with Ashley, when she was just three years old. I was participating in ectoparasitic research projects

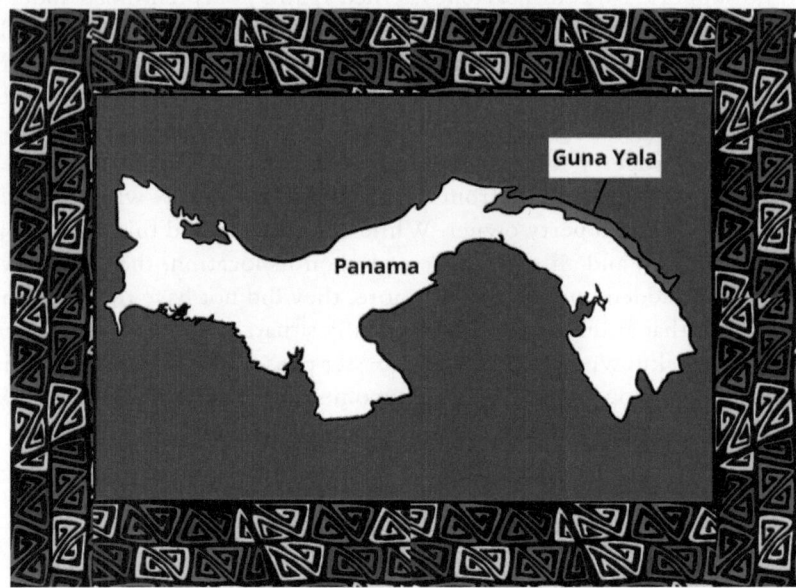

FIGURE 2.1 Comarca de Guna Yala, Panama. Designed by Sophia Mohammad,
February 2021.

related to scabies and headlice. I had been working there since the 1980s,
so the community members were very eager to meet my young daughter
(Figure 2.1). Comarca de Guna Yala, Panama.
Ashley enjoyed the freedom to play with the children in an uncompli-
cated island surrounded by homes with thatched roofs, simple outhouses,
sandy streets, and no paved roads or cars to avoid. It didn't matter that
she could not speak the native *Guna* language. With her pale skin and
blue eyes, they affectionately called her *sipu*, meaning albino. Albinos are
very common in the Guna Yala population, which has one of the highest
albinism rates in the world.

The history of albino Gunas is well documented in the literature. The
genetic trait and intermarriage are key contributing factors, with the first
reference of albinism dated back to 1640, noting "there were many who
were white and blond as flemings,"[33] so Ashley fit right in. Guna mothers
do their best to protect their albino children from the harsh tropical sun
and extreme heat that causes many health problems to both their sensitive
eyes and unpigmented skin. Their access to sunscreen and sunglasses,
while available in the cities, was limited on the remote island.

We would always bring these requested supplies for the albino community health worker, Alonzo Brenes, so he could distribute throughout

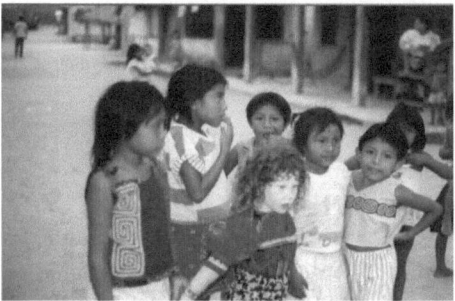

FIGURE 2.2   Ashley with Guna Friends in 1991. By author.

the community. Alonzo did then, and continues today, to provide health education to his community. As a community leader, and *vocero* (spokesperson) for their *congreso* (gathering house), he teaches families about protecting their albino children with hats, sunscreen, and sunglasses, and to keep them indoors during the day as much as possible. I learned that bringing supplies was not the best practice for sustainable public health actions, and the local- and national-level government would soon need to take a greater role in protecting this vulnerable population.

Of course, everyone wanted to play with Ashley, the *sipu waga* (albino foreigner) (Figure 2.2).

Lessons for All

My three-year-old daughter's first international experience occurred in the Guna village of Ticantiki/Niadub, which had a total population of 756 in 1991. Today, the population is just over 1,000 people. Ashley mimicked the other children's activities, as all young kids tend to do. The older girls wanted to carry her and tote her on their hips, as you would see older siblings do throughout the village. I monitored her closely to avoid sharing her small hairbrush or playing with the pretty hair bows. Headlice was endemic, and the crawling creatures will hunt for a new head of hair to lay their eggs and multiply. Using a comb on her child's head, a mother removed some of the lice and eggs, also known as nits. I showed Ashley the lice, the tiny crawling bugs, and she made the yucky face, suggesting she understood. Seeing is believing, which is a valuable public health educational tool.

I was less successful in getting Ashley to keep her shoes on when many, or most, of the children did not use shoes to play in. For the older children, the good shoes were reserved for school. I had to use my best parenting skills with her because I already knew that kids like to fit in and not feel different from others. I recall telling her that some of the children may be poor and did not own shoes, and that is why they were often sick.

I was not able to show her the parasites in sand, nor the worms that could enter her body through dirty hands or unprotected feet and migrate to compete for nutrition, ultimately causing a distended belly full of worms to flourish. I already knew about the public health challenges in getting older children and adults to understand parasitic infestations, so I had to remain vigilant, while she continued to fight.

"No shoes, no shoes," she insisted.

It was two years later when I realized that the continual battle to keep her shoes on may have had a lasting impression, whether appropriately aimed or not. We were visiting a farmworker community in South Florida in December to deliver holiday gifts to the children through a program called *Mujeres Unidas en Justica, Educacion, y Reforma* (MUJER – Women United in Justice, Education and Reform). Ashley, then five years old, had a puzzled look on her face. I explained that the families were too poor to buy their children holiday gifts and they needed their money for food, housing, and school supplies. She leaned over and said, "But mommy, these children aren't poor. Look, they're all wearing shoes." Her perception of poverty was shaped by her earlier experiences.

Conclusion

Researchers will criticize individual observations as unscientific methods. Yet we know that having different observations about a situation can influence the point of departure one takes in research. Interestingly, the notion of measuring shoes worn can actually be a useful indicator for economic progress, public health, and development.

It reminds me of a story recounted by Hans Rosling during a meeting with the Prime Minister of Mozambique in 2002.[34] The Prime Minister said he didn't need to look at their gross domestic product to make an assessment on their economic progress. Rather, he observed the shoes worn during the annual May marches when everyone was dressed their very best. The entire population would be out marching; therefore, no one could borrow shoes. He looked to see who had new shoes, old shoes, or were barefoot. He then compared this to what he observed the previous year,[35] not necessarily scientific, yet very insightful and important to understanding how individuals form their opinions and create different perspectives.

This is a good lesson. We need to take more time and listen to another's perspective. This applies to first impressions, as a young child, or as leader's knowledge about the livelihoods and well-being of the people they serve. It seems instinctive to me that researchers and community health programs would include more input from the different stakeholders and embrace the viewpoints of children and leaders before they settle upon their own first impressions.

Ashley arrived with two pairs of shoes on her first trip to Guna Yala, Panama. As it was no surprise, she left one pair for another young child to keep. Clearly, the understanding of poverty extends beyond the topic of shoes. It provides a starting point. First experiences shape our perspectives and I suggest this requires further inquiry.

Concluding Remarks

The relationship of public health, poverty, inequality, and development is a good starting point to advance the study of population health. It exposes the inextricable ties that public health has to the wider political, social, cultural, economic, environmental, ecological conditions and consequential policies.

In conclusion, I do not want to minimize the increasing impact of development and noncommunicable diseases such as cancers, coronary heart and vascular diseases, and diabetes. This will be discussed in the proceeding chapter on globalization and public health.

Notes

1 Organisation for Economic Co-operation and Development and The World Bank, *Health at a Glance: Latin America and the Caribbean 2020* (Paris: OECD Publishing, 2020), doi:10.1787/6089164f-en.
2 United Nations Development Programme, *2018 Statistical Update: Human Development Indices and Indicators* (New York: UNDP, 2018), http://hdr.undp.org/en/2018-update.
3 United Nations Development Programme and the Oxford Poverty and Human Development Initiative, *Global Multidimensional Poverty Index 2019: Illuminating Inequalities* (UNDP & OPHI, 2019), http://hdr.undp.org/en/2019-MPI.
4 Amaryta Sen, *Development as Freedom* (New York: Alfred A Knopf, 1999).
5 See "Multidimensional Poverty Index: Developing Countries, Table 1," http://hdr.undp.org/sites/default/files/mpi_2019_table_1.pdf.
6 Marta Alanis and Jacqueline Nolley Echegaray, "Fighting for Women's Lives in Argentina: Making the Connection between Abortion Rights, Human Rights and People Power," *Conscience* 32, no. 3 (2011): 29.
7 Melissa Rosenstein, G. Romero, and Mariana Ramos, "Maternal Mortality in Argentina: A Closer Look at Women Who Die Outside of the Health System," *Maternal and Child Health Journal* 12, no. 4 (2008): 519–524.

8 Theories of modernization, dependency, and world systems analysis offer historical and structural considerations about the social, cultural, and economic determinants of population inequalities within and across countries in Latin America and the Caribbean. While a more in-depth discussion is beyond the scope of this book, some selected books are included in the bibliography at the end of the chapter.

9 Asa Cristina Laurell, "Editorial: Lasting Lessons from Social Ideas and Movements of the Sixties on Latin American Public Health," *American Journal of Public Health* 108, no. 6 (June 2018): 731.

10 Deepa Narayan and Patti Petesch, *Voices of the Poor: From Many Lands* (Washington, DC: World Bank and Oxford University Press, 2002), http://hdl.handle.net/10986/14053.

11 See both Robert Chamber, *Rural Development: Putting the Last First* (New York: Routledge, 1983, and Commission on Health Research for Development, "Health and Development," in *Health Research: Essential Link to Equity in Development*, eds. John Evans et al. (Oxford: Oxford University Press, 1990), 11.

12 Peter Hotez, *Blue Marble Health: An Innovative Plan to Fight Disease of the Poor and Wealth* (Baltimore, MD: Johns Hopkins University Press, 2016), 11.

13 See Centers for Disease Control and Prevention, with 70 million, accessed November 2019, https://www.cdc.gov/parasites/chagas/gen_info/detailed.html#intro, and Pan American Health Organization, accessed November 2019, https://www.paho.org/en/topics/chagas-disease.

14 Margaret Chan, "Return to Alma-Ata," *The Lancet* 372, no. 9642 (September 2008): 866.

15 See Jerry M. Spiegel, Jaime Breilh, and Annalee Yassi, "Why Language Matters: Insights and Challenges in Applying a Social Determination of Health Approach in a North-South Collaborative Research Program," *Globalization and Health* 11, no. 9 (2015): 2, doi: 10.1186/s12992-015-0091-2; Rafael Gonzalez Guzmán, "Latin American Social Medicine and the Report of the WHO Commission on Social Determinants of Health," *Social Medicine* 4 (2009): 113–120; and Centro Brasileiro de Estudos de Saúde, *Determinação Social da Saúde e Reforma Sanitária* (Rio de Janeiro: CEBES, 2010).

16 Vicente Navarro, "Determinants of Health: What We Mean by Social Determinants of Health," *International Journal of Health Sciences* 39, no. 3 (2009): 440.

17 Carissa F. Etienne, "Achieving Social Equity," in *'To Save Humanity': What Matters Most for a Health Future*, eds. Julio Frenk and Steven Hoffman (Oxford: Oxford University Press, 2015), 107–108.

18 Alicia Bárcena, United Nations Economic Commission on Latin America and the Caribbean (UN ECLAC), "Addressing Inequalities and Challenges to Social Inclusion through Fiscal, Wage and Social Protections Policies," (Presentation, 57th Session of the Commission for Social Development, United Nations Headquarters, NY, February 13, 2009).

19 World Bank Group, "The World Bank approves US $100 million to combat malnutrition in Guatemala," *Press Release*, March 27, 2017, https://www.worldbank.org/en/news/press-release/2017/03/27/the-world-bank-approves-us100-million-to-combat-malnutrition-in-guatemala.

20 Global Financing Facility, *Country Spotlight: Guatemala*, https://www.globalfinancingfacility.org/sites/gff_new/files/Guatemala_EN_Web.pdf.

21 World Bank Group, "The World Bank approves US $100 million to combat malnutrition in Guatemala," *Press Release*, March 27, 2017, https://www.worldbank.org/en/news/press-release/2017/03/27/the-world-bank-approves-us100-million-to-combat-malnutrition-in-guatemala.

22 Global Financing Facility, *Crecer Sano, Cruzada Nacional por la Nutrición, Gobierno de la República de Guatemala 2020–2024*, https://www.globalfinancingfacility. org/sites/gff_new/files/documents/Guatemala-Investment-Case-Cruzada-Nacional-por-la-Nutricion_ES.pdf.

23 Pan American Health Organization, *Necesidad Prioritaria de Salud en Centro América y Panamá* (documento báscio) (San Jose, CA and Costa Rica: PAHO, 1984).

24 Pan American Health Organization, *Health Conditions in the Americas, 1980–1984*, 2 vols. (Washington, DC: PAHO, 1986).

25 Latin America Caribbean Regional Office, *Poverty in Latin America: The Impact of Depression* (Report 6389) (Washington, DC: The World Bank, 1986).

26 Philip Musgrove, "The Economic Crisis and Its Impact on Health Care in Latin America and the Caribbean," *International Journal of Health Services* 17, no. 3 (1987): 411–441.

27 Jose Carlos Escuedro, "Los Sistemas de Informacion en Salud en America Latina," *Revista Centroamericana de Ciencias de la Salud* 5, no. 14 (1979): 109–122.

28 Giovanni Andrea Cornia, Richard Jolly, and Frances Stewart, eds., *Adjustment with a Human Face: Protecting the Vulnerable and Promoting Growth* (Oxford: Oxford University Press, 1987).

29 UNICEF, "The Americas and Caribbean Regional Office and the Regional Programme Women in Development," *The Invisible Adjustment: Poor Women and the Economic Crisis* (Santiago: UNICEF, 1989).

30 Asa Cristina Laurell, "What Does Latin American Social Medicine Do When It Governs? The Case Study of Mexico City Government," *American Journal of Public Health* 9, no. 12 (December 2001): 2028.

31 Declaration of Alma Ata, International Conference on Primary Health Care, Alma Ata, Russia, September 6–12, 1978. See Section VI: https://www.who.int/ publications/almaata_declaration_en.pdf.

32 The Commission on Social Determinants of Health final report emphasized that health needs to be reviewed in all government policies. See Margaret Chan, "Return to Alma-Ata," *The Lancet* 372, no. 9642 (September 2008).

33 D.B. Stout, "Further Notes on Albinism among the San Blas, Cuna, Panama," *American Journal of Physical Anthropology* 4, no. 4 (December 1946): 483. See also Juan Requejo Salcedo, "Relación histórica y geográfica de la provincia de Panamá (1640)," in *Colección de libros y documentos referentes á la historia de América*, vol. 8 (Madrid, 1908).

34 Hans Rosling with Ola Rosling and Ana Rosling Rönnlund, *Factfulness: Ten Reasons We're Wrong about the World – And Why Things Are Better than You Think* (New York: Flatiron Books, 2018). Note: Renowned global health physician and statistician, Hans Rosling, Hans Rosling passed away February 7, 2017.

35 Ibid., 191–192.

Bibliography – Selected Books

Beaglehole, Robert. *Global Public Health: A New Era*. Oxford: Oxford University Press, 2003.

Cardoso, Fernando Henrique and Faletto, Enzo. *Dependency and Development in Latin America*, trans. Majory Mattingly Urquidi. Berkeley: University of California Press, 1979.

Cornia, Giovanni, Andrea, Jolly, Richard and Steward, Frances, eds. *Adjustment with a Human Face: Protecting the Vulnerable and Promoting Growth*. Oxford: Oxford University Press, 1987.

Gatti, Anna and Boggio, Andrea, eds. *Health and Development*. New York: Palgrave Macmillan, 2009.

Glassman, Amanda and Temin, Miriam. *Millions Saved – New Cases of Proven Success in Global Health*. Washington, DC: Center for Global Development, 2016.

Farmer, Paul. *Infections and Inequalities. The Modern Plagues*. Oakland: University of California Press, 1999.

Farmer, Paul. *Pathologies of Power. Health, Human Rights and the War on the Poor*. Oakland: University of California Press, 2003.

Foster, George M. *Traditional Cultures and The impact of Technology Change*. New York: Harper & Row, 1962.

Frank, Andre Gunder. *Capitalism and Underdevelopment in Latin America*. New York: New York University Press, 1967.

Hotez, Peter J. *Blue Marble Health: An Innovative Plan to fight Disease of the Poor Amid Wealth*. Baltimore, MD: Johns Hopkins University, 2016.

Levine, Ruth. *Case Studies in Global Health: Millions Saved*. Burlington, VT: Jones and Bartlett Publishers. 2007.

Newell, Kenneth, ed. *Health by the People*. Switzerland: World Health Organization, 1975.

Navarro, Vicente and Muntaner, Carles. *Political and Economic Determinants of Population Health and Well-being- Controversies and Development*. New York: Routledge, 2004.

Navarro, Vicente, ed. *Imperialism, Health and Medicine*. New York: Baywood Publishing Company, Inc, 1979.

Prebisch, Raúl. *Change and Development-Latin Americas Great Task: Report Submitted to the InterAmerican Development Bank*. New York: Praeger Publishers, 1971.

Rodriguez-Garcia Rosalie and Goldman, Ann, eds. *The Health-Development Link*. Washington, DC: Pan American Health Organization, 1994.

Rosling, Hans, Rosing, Ola, and Rosling Rönnlund, Ana. *Factfulness: Ten Reasons We're Wrong About the World-And Why Things Are Better Than You Think*. New York: Flatiron Books, 2018.

Sachs, Jeffery D. *Macroeconomics and Health: Investing in Health for Economic Development*. Report of the Commission on Macroeconomics and Health. Geneva: World Health Organization. 2001.

Sen, Amartya K. *Development as Freedom*. New York: Alfred A Knopf, Random House 1999.

Wallerstein, Immanuel. *The Modern World-System 1: Capitalist Agriculture and the Origins of the European World Economy in the Sixteenth Century*. New York: Academic Press, 1974.

3
GLOBALIZATION AND PUBLIC HEALTH

The first time I thought about globalization and public health was not about the spread of a highly infectious disease across borders. Curiously, in 1982 a barge stacked high with cases of Coca-Cola navigated by me along the Magdalena River in Colombia. I was traveling from Barrancabermeja, located in the northern central part of the country, to the Casaba Shell Colombia, S.A. oil fields situated in the isolated areas along the middle of the Magdalena River. This took place before I knew about the historic importance of the river, which has been an essential transportation route for this Andean region. The Magdalena River connects the interior cities of Colombia with the Caribbean Sea. Nevertheless, the character of the river is best known through the eyes of Gabriel García Márquez in two of his famous works, *Love in the Time of Cholera (1985)*, and *The General in His Labyrinth (1989)* (Figure 3.1).

I thought it was remarkable that Coca-Cola could market their products to the most remote communities. Why couldn't public health prevention strategies work in the same way? It could not. Unless, of course, Coke products were offered to encourage participation in a community health education program. This presents the paradox of public health and business, then and now.

After that encounter, I learned about the term coca colonization, which describes how the globalization of American culture, and products such as Coca-Cola, created new consumption and behavior changes as an illustration of American capitalism. Some called it American cultural imperialism, while others argued it was the inevitable outcome of a worldwide shift toward cultural hybridization. As you will read in this chapter, the rising consumption of American sugar sweet beverages and processed dense foods arriving in Latin America and the Caribbean has created substantial changes in the drinking,

DOI: 10.4324/9781003007401-4

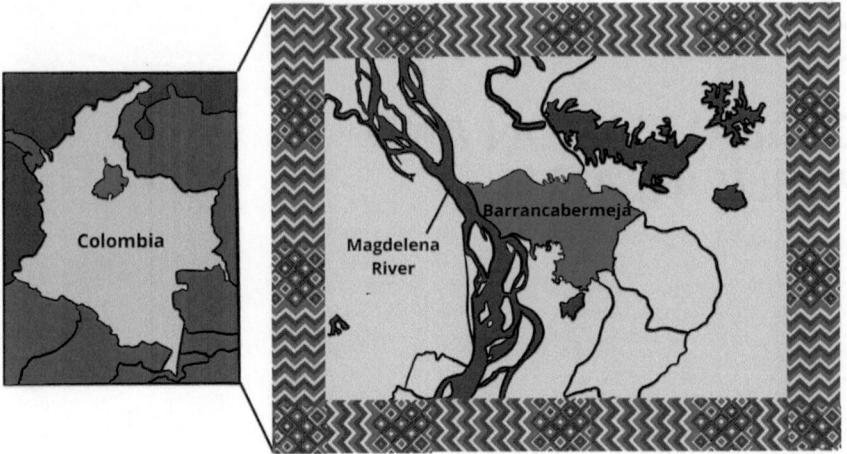

FIGURE 3.1 Magdalena River, Barrancabermeja, Colombia. Design and Artwork by Sofia Mohammad, February 2021.

eating, and nutritional patterns across the region, contributing to what is referred to as the epidemiologic, health, and nutritional transitions.

Most globalization studies have centered around the economic factors; however, more recent research has drawn its attention to the direct and indirect impacts globalization has on public health consequences. With the boundaries of human interactions and exchanges of goods, services, and intensification of sharing information, there has been a call for more rigorous study on trade, foreign direct investments, and public health. Specific examples and closer examination of case studies in Latin America and the Caribbean will show how both communicable and noncommunicable diseases are closely linked to globalization, with positive and negative outcomes.

The historical perspectives on the spread of infectious diseases in the Americas, from the arrival of smallpox to mosquito-borne diseases such as yellow fever, malaria, and dengue fever, are all associated with further and faster trade and travel. However, evidence on epidemiologic, health, and nutritional transitions illustrates how the rapidly rising noncommunicable diseases such as cancers, heart disease, diabetes, and obesity within poor and middle-income countries in the region also requires more attention. The relationship of chronic diseases to globalization, trade, and foreign direct investments has lagged behind the more obvious linkages with epidemics and pandemics related to infectious diseases.

The study of globalization and public health requires a broader understanding beyond the economic well-being to include the social, cultural, political, environmental, ecological, and technological factors. In doing this, scrutinizing the unequal influences of globalization and public health from a subpopulation, national, regional, or global level has taken an important path of study. While praising globalization as the opportunity to have more access to information, services, or goods, it is useful to explore how such interactions may also present negative public health consequences with unequal outcomes. The benefit of having improved public health information, new drugs or treatments, is juxtaposed to having more exposure to new pathogens, sugary drinks, fast foods, tobacco products, and other unhealthy practices. Also, such commodities may not benefit all equally, and for many in Latin America and the Caribbean this remains a reality. It means little to a rural poor household in Honduras that dire poverty has declined globally, as India and China continue along a path of economic growth with rising trade and foreign direct investment opportunities. The role globalization plays, and how it shapes public health outcomes, is an important question, with no simple answer.

From post-World War II through the end of the Cold War in 1991, Latin America saw increasing social democracy which emerged from Europe's 19th-century struggle of labor and money. The rise of "Christian democracy" spread from Venezuela to Chile, El Salvador, Guatemala, Costa Rica, and Mexico. This corresponded with ideologies to promote more equitable distribution of income and investments in social protection programs, which supported improved public health outcomes. So why is Latin America so unequal today, with evidence of rich and poor health disparities throughout the region? One way to examine this is through an analysis of neoliberal policies of trade and globalization, albeit, not the sole explanation. It is instructive to recognize the different terms of globalization and the direct and indirect relationships to population health. Globalization may have started well before the term was first used in the mid-1940s, gaining the momentum with the business sector in late 1980s to expand its further reach today. It could be argued that the earliest stage of globalization started along the Silk Road trading route during the 1st century BC when trade expanded from local and regional exchange of goods to a global endeavor.

Globalization Terms

Globalization is defined in many ways with language as interconnectedness; integration; homogenization; intensification; deterritorialization and planetary connections; expansion; or the hybridization in the flow of goods, services, people, microbes and diseases, ideas, values, and behaviors across borders. There is no shortage of viewpoints about the benefits and detriments of globalization.

International relations scholars, Robert Keohane and Joseph Nye, explain globalization as networks creating greater interdependence and interconnectedness across people, ideas, and information, with the importance of environmental and biological factors. Such increasing flows and influences of globalization are important to understanding how this impacts population health. David

Held, another international relations scholar and political scientist, explored the faster, further, and deeper levels of interconnectedness requiring a closer examination of the underlying factors. Stephen Gilpin presents another international relations viewpoint about the increasing integration between trade and economics as this relationship continues to intensify. He proposes a better understanding of the political and social relationships of nation-states, which extend beyond the economic factors. Joseph Stiglitz, Noble Prize in Economics expanded upon the role that international financial institutions and world trade regimes play in globalization. In his 2002 book, *Globalization and Its Discontents*, Stiglitz concentrated his attention on the International Monetary Fund and World Bank's roles specifically, with consideration of the World Trade Organization (WTO). Roland Robertson was a pioneering sociologist to apply the term globalization in 2002 and theorized that as the intensification and compression of the world was underway so was a shared consciousness about how we view the world. Ethan Kapstein, political economist, examines government's role in responding to the economic and political consequences of globalization since the post-WWII era. Susan Strange, another international relations scholar, is best known for her work on globalization, corporate influence, and pedagogical leadership for the study of international political economy. Her focus on money and power shaping global markets contributed to more recent areas of study in public health associated with applied research on the CDoH. The rise of corporate power and such influence over economics and world politics since WWII have made some large corporations more powerful than smaller states. This is seen today with the shift from state-state conflicts to disputes of powerful multinational corporations against states, which will be presented in an example about the tobacco industry in Uruguay.

Jan Scholte, a European international development scholar, presents the view of the increasing porosity of state sovereignty across the social, economic, and political factors that traverse borders. His argument on increasing transplanetary connections offers important insights into the nexus of globalization and public health in contemporary times. Sociologist Anthony Giddens emphasizes the intensification of social interactions through global connections, which help shape local behaviors. Both Strange and Giddens discuss the increased influence of global corporations and their economic power and political sway. Thomas Friedman, a three-time Pulitzer Prize author, reporter, and columnist, suggests that globalization requires a more robust study on the integration between states, markets, and technology, with the increasing reach of information systems and telecommunications. A perspective associated with cultural hybridization, a term coined by Argentine anthropologist, Nestor Garcia-Candin, offers important insights into globalization in Latin America. His work examines cultural homogenization associated with globalization, media, arts, and the diffusion of customs, ideas, and behaviors attributable to the erosion of physical space and territories. These definitions, while not intended to be an exhaustive list, reveal the interconnectedness of globalization and public health as we explore the increasing role of trade, travel, tourism, and the exchange of information, ideas, and principles.

While there is no standard language for globalization, there is an agreed upon term for health. The universally accepted term coined by the World Health (1948) is the state of complete physical, social, and mental well-being and not merely the absence of disease or infirmity. It was Sir Donald Acheson's report to the United Kingdom in 1988[1] helped refine an agreement on public health as the "art and science of preventing disease, prolonging life, promoting health through organized efforts of society," which underscores the collective action to achieve, secure, and maintain population well-being. Subsequently, the association of globalization and public health can be better realized with the clarity of terms.

In Chapters 1 and 2, we discussed the significance of the social determinants of health, and in this chapter, we will expand the discussion to include the CDoH. The CDoH correspond to how corporations may have a negative effect on population health, including such terms as profit-driven diseases, corporate-induced diseases, unhealthy commodities, vectors of disease, and industrial epidemics to name some of the language used with the rising rates of noncommunicable diseases in low- and middle-income countries (LMICs). Gerald Hastings argued for more research on marketing tactics and the use of corporate power that could produce unhealthy practices and poor health outcomes.[2] John Millar presented the term commercial determinants to show how there are both good and bad corporations; therefore, he argues, it is the government's responsibility to protect population health and the environment from such industries that are harmful.[3] The positive side is businesses provide employment opportunities, tax revenues, and contribute to economic development, while the negative impact has wider implications for population health and the planet.[4] Iona Kickbush et al. present a conceptual framework to stimulate further discussion about the commercial determinants, starting with identifying the drivers of internationalization of trade, demand for growth, and the expanding outreach of corporations. They propose that through the channels of marketing, supply chain, lobbying, and corporate citizenship, businesses have an impact on population health and the environment.[5] Melissa Mailon et al. illustrate how corporate political activity within the study of the CDoH has influenced public health in Colombia through an interrelationship of government, food industry, and the media. In the first study conducted in Latin America to assess corporate political activity in the food industry, researchers documented business involvement in the scientific evidence on diet and nutrition, their participation in decision making, and ultimately how they influenced public policy.[6]

The history of globalization and population health, which is rooted in the issue of transborder spread of infectious diseases, has expanded to include the larger concerns for planetary health. Nevertheless, it is equally important to reflect upon the positive influences of corporate investments in host countries. Transnational corporations may contribute to economic growth, offer employment opportunities, and increase access to markets. Taxation revenues from corporate investments may improve services to promote population welfare such as health and education. Furthermore, the rise in both social corporate responsibility and social movements to confront the social, environmental, economic, and population health concerns through shared values places public and private partnerships at the crossroads of globalization and public health.

History of Globalization and Public Health

The focus on controlling the spread of diseases from the East to the West has historically been framed within the economic interests and the ability to carry out commerce. I maintain this may be no different in contemporary times. The history of human movements, from travel, migration, and conquest, tells the story of how the wider human interactions and movements have exchanged microbes. From the first pandemic plague of Justinian in the Byzantine Empire from 542 AD to the 1370 Black Plague quarantine of ships, knowledge about the spread of diseases continued to advance. It is not only human migration but also nonhumans such as birds who also are natural hosts for many arboviruses, where the spread of diseases and transfer of viruses from animal to human are referred to as zoonotic diseases. Research today suggests that approximately 70–80% of all new human infectious diseases originated in animals and jump species to infect humans, presenting as a spillover event.

The 14th-century quarantine practices in Europe made significant contributions to modern-day public health. Prior to the 1700s we observed a population shift to more temperate climates and modifying lifestyles. The migration to the Americas brought along the unwelcomed gifts of deadly microorganisms to this hemisphere. The historical shame of African slaves and colonizers bringing smallpox, malaria, and yellow fever, contributing to the rapid population decline in the Americas, characterizes the transfer of microbes across the globe. History also reveals how the dual decimation, the murderous acts and the spread of infectious diseases, wreaked havoc on the native populations who were never previously unexposed to measles, German measles, mumps, plague, chicken pox, and trachoma (a bacterial infection of the eyes). It wasn't until 1971 that a combined vaccine for measles, mumps, and rubella (German measles), known as MMR, was available. Before that people continued to suffer or die, especially the young children.

Earlier shifts of populations and exposures to new germs are an important piece of the global public health puzzle. It shows how prior eras of globalization have been a part of the population health history and exposes its ugly side in the Americas. During the 20th century, in the Western Hemisphere, the intensification of globalization created more unequal relationships, dispropor-tionate health outcomes, and yet, limited study was conducted until recently. We know how the Industrial Revolution era paved the way for a dramatic increase in travel, trade, and the spread of pathogens all aligning with the de-velopment of steamships in the early 1800s and the railroad boom later that century. The construction of the Suez Canal connecting the Mediterranean Sea to the Red Sea (1869) and the completion of the Panama Canal with pas-sage across the Atlantic to the Pacific (1914) provided the route for quicker and further reach of people, goods, and microbes. Microorganisms do not require a passport; they can sneak aboard a boat, train, or plane hiding among the arriv-ing goods or attack an unsuspecting victim. It can happen through exposures to contaminated water, food (animal, plant, or tree), air, environment, or a fomite such as utensils, personal items, or other goods.

Early Trade and Health

The spread of diseases related to trade has historically been a contentious battle between the protection of commerce and trade and the protection of public health. The *Conseil Superieur de la Santé* (Superior Council of Health) was estab-lished in 1838 in Constantinople with key maritime states from the Ottoman Empire to prevent the cross-border spread of deadly communicable diseases such as cholera and plague. This was the world's first-known nongovernmental or-ganization network formed to tackle issues beyond borders that were previously left to nation-states to respond on their own. The implementation of quarantine across countries required a joint action and cooperation. Interestingly, "... a sov-ereign state would allow an international administration to control these matters on its territory can only be explained by the existing political relationships"[7] in which the Ottoman Empire was weakening with greater dependency on mar-itime states. Was it the fear of the spread of plague and cholera's impact on the people, or the protection of commerce, or both that motivated such international health collaboration? Does it have to be approached as a dichotomy? We know that answer, and here we are in 2020 faced with the same questions in the midst of the Severe acute respiratory syndrome coronavirus (SARS-CoV-2) pandemic.

The Middle Ages posed many health threats and epidemics in European cities as the population grew and water, sanitation, housing posed many hy-gienic risks to the population. Not knowing the causes of the diseases, it was observed that detaining ships for 40 days would reduce the spread of cholera or plague. Quarantine meaning 40 in Italian, and along with the French term *cordon sanitaire,* restricting the movement of people or goods in a de-fined area as a way to stop the spread of infectious diseases, established early public health prevention strategies. Lessons from history show how during the late 1300s a 30-day period of isolation was used to prevent the spread of diseases. There are many rationales for why 40 days. It could be that 30 days was insufficient time to stop the spread of diseases. Or it could be related to biblical times for the 40 days it took Moses to reach Mount Sinai to receive the Ten Commandments.

The earlier exchange of goods produced both positive and negative outcomes, as detailed in the work of Giovanni Berlinguer, where he presents a non-Eurocentric approach to emphasize the *mutuo descrubrimiento* (mutual discovery) of reciprocal contributions of the old and new world.[8] The interchange and diffusion of infectious diseases from syphilis to malaria and yellow fever have been documented throughout history with disagreements about the origin of syphilis. This unmasks the stigmatization of many infectious diseases, especially those that are sexually transmitted. History is replete with examples blaming populations for a disease outbreak. While Germany, Italy, and the United Kingdom called syphilis the French disease, the French called it the Neapolitan Disease. It was Girolamo Fracastoro, Italian physician, poet, whose research on the transmission of syphilis in the 1500s that could be the early start of epidemiology. He conceptualized how epidemic diseases were caused by germs; however, this was not scientifically validated until 300 years later through the research of French microbiologist, Louis Pasteur.

Berlinguer[9] also conveys the outcomes of international exchanges such as exotic foods, plants, and their impact on health and nutrition, as well as drug addiction. The export of fruits, vegetables, and roots from the Americas to Europe contributed to the improvements in health with better nutrition in the West. Yet, exchanges of deadly microbes also caused the potato blight in the 1840s. Potatoes, first cultivated thousands of years ago in Peru and Bolivia, were exported to Europe in the 1500s and became a dominant feature of the Irish diet. The Irish became dependent upon cultivating and consuming potatoes, so when the potato blight struck Ireland, increased malnutrition, starvation, and disease caused more than 1 million deaths. In 2016, scientists using ancient DNA discovered that the origin of the Irish Potato Famine was caused by a fungus-like microorganism, *phytophthora infestans*, originally identified in South America.[10]

Other crop exchanges, such as the production and consumption of coca in Peru and Bolivia, played an important part of profitable trade historically and continues today through illicit drug trade.

Throughout history, trade and migration disputes have brought attention to the transborder spread of diseases, which virologist Stephen Morse refers to as microbial or viral trafficking. This spread has been facilitated by the scientific advancements in transportation, of which the tracing of movements can be associated with better travel routes.

Modern-day restrictions in regional or global trade from the 1991 cholera outbreak in Peru to the wider fear from SARS in 2003 showed the interconnectedness of public health, economics, and commerce. A May 2003 World Health Organization (WHO) press release reported, our experience with SARS is the firm link between health, trade, tourism, and commerce. If they didn't see it before, Presidents, Prime Ministers and Finance and Trade Ministers, are now seeing first-hand the impact of health on the economic, social and political fabric of nations.

Public health crosses all sectors of society and requires collective action. After almost a century free of cholera in Latin America and the Caribbean, it re-emerged in Peru in 1991. Towns along the Peruvian coast, with strong trade relations with Asian countries, suffered the greatest impact of cholera, spreading throughout the entire northern coast of Peru in ten days.[11] The closing of the international markets to Peruvian products caused great concerns since the fishing industry that employed more than 56,000 Peruvians and the trade and tourism industries estimated losses from cholera at $770 million.[12]

Globalization and Smallpox

There are many examples to show the relationship of globalization and the spread of infectious diseases throughout the Americas. One of the earliest examples is smallpox, which remains the only know human disease to ever be eradicated. While other examples will be discussed in this chapter, case studies will be further developed in the chapter on health diplomacy to demonstrate regional cooperation to prevent, detect, and control diseases in Latin America and the Caribbean.

The spread of smallpox is one of the earliest portrayals of a deadly disease traversing the globe. Rapid transportation, population growth, urbanization, science and technology, agricultural and manufacturing, and expanding trade routes are all contributing factors that facilitated quicker and further movements of people and goods. Smallpox is a highly infectious virus spread through sneezing, coughing air droplet, or open scabs, which seep fluid. According to the Centers for Disease Control and Prevention (CDC), smallpox-like rashes were found in mummies dated back to the 3rd-century BCE Egyptian Empire. The history of smallpox shows the earliest description of the disease was identified in the 4th-century CE China, and its origin remains unknown. It found its way to Europe during the 5th and 7th centuries with large deaths tolls during the Middle Ages.[13]

We know smallpox reached the Americas when Spanish conquistadors and African slaves arrived in the Western Hemisphere in 1507. Smallpox wreaked havoc killing entire tribes, creeping through the island of Hispaniola. Native Americans continued to die as it spread further to Cuba in a little over a decade, reaching Puerto Rico the following year and killing more than half of the population. According to historian William McNeill, when Cuban ships arrived to Mexico in 1519, the population was reduced from 25 million to 1.6 million in just over one century because of the deadly smallpox virus. The decimation of Aztecs to the Incas in Peru in 1524 was followed by further deaths of Brazil's populations within a few decades. By the 1580s smallpox was widespread throughout South America, where port cities continued to serve as epidemic hubs for the disease. The greatest smallpox toll took place in the Caribbean where native population were replaced by African slaves and Spanish settlers. The belief in the god of smallpox, Shapona, also referred to as King of the Earth, Obaluaye, was considered god's displeasure with the people. Such beliefs were practiced among the Yoruba in West Africa and brought to Haiti, Cuba, and Bahia, Brazil with the African slaves. Consequently, recognizing the social, cultural, and religious influences, which impact how prevention, control, and treatment interventions are implemented across populations, is as important then as it is in contemporary times. Interventions to control the spread of diseases are not always uniform, as a country or region of the Western Hemisphere grapples to adapt methods and strategies that are culturally relevant and respect local norms.

It was an English scientist and physician, Edward Jenner, who developed the smallpox vaccine in 1779. He observed that dairymaids who became infected with a milder disease from cowpox were not victimized by the affliction of smallpox. He extracted fluid from a dairymaid's cowpox sore to inoculate his own gardener's nine-year-old son. The child developed only mild symptoms for a few days. Two months later Jenner inoculated this same young boy with lesions from an active smallpox case but he did not get the disease. Jenner concluded that he was protected by this inoculation. Clearly, these would be highly unethical research practices today, but this paved the way for the field of immunology and eventually the acceptance and development of a smallpox vaccine.

Smallpox remained a public health challenge. In the 1950s the Pan American Sanitary Bureau (PASB) implemented a regional eradication campaign to stop the scourge of smallpox, with the successful elimination of the disease across Mexico, Peru, Venezuela, and Colombia. In 1961, the PASB documented that 70% of the cases were occurring in Brazil and 22% in Ecuador, with other countries reporting smaller percentage of cases. Nevertheless, it was the ambitious global campaign under the leadership of the WHO and the rigor of the regional office, Pan American Sanitation Organization in 1966, that countries in Latin America became free of smallpox. It took eight years from the start of the campaign, with Brazil and Argentina becoming the last two countries to report no new cases or transmission throughout the Western Hemisphere.

There have been other infectious diseases eliminated from Latin American and the Caribbean countries or brought under a manageable control; however, in 1980 smallpox became the first known human disease to be eradicated, meaning there are no more cases anywhere around the world. It is important to acknowledge that smallpox is not extinct since stockpiles of the virus are housed in high-level security laboratories in the United States and Russia. Smallpox remains a Class A biological agent, a high-level pathogen considered as a potential weapon of bioterrorism. Post-9/11 U.S. military troops have been vaccinated as part of a U.S. national program of preparedness against biological weapons.[14]

The smallpox vaccine was widely accepted then, while today we observe an increase in vaccine hesitancy and the rise in anti-vaxxer movements as a contributing factor to the re-emergence of vaccine preventable diseases. Researchers in Latin America and the Caribbean call for a better understanding of this issue by using the WHO's Strategic Advisory Group of Experts Model of Determinants of Vaccine Hesitancy based on three factors: confidence, complacency, and convenience of vaccine. In a recent study, Guzman-Holtz et al. stated that no systematic reviews in Latin America and the Caribbean have been conducted to identify the key barriers to vaccination.[15] While there is no simplistic answer, when populations refuse a vaccine for religious, lifestyle, or other rationales, herd immunity may not have been met and the spread will threaten unprotected and susceptible populations, including the very young, old, immunocompromised populations such as those receiving chemotherapy or living with AIDS should be untreated for HIV/AIDS. This is especially important for measles since it requires 90–95% of the population to be vaccinated to reach herd immunity. It is no surprise that with increased globalization, population shifts, and displacement this is becoming more of a challenge to prevent and protect populations. We are currently in the middle of the worst pandemic in over a century, with estimates that 60–80% herd immunity will be necessary to protect populations to prevent further spread; yet, there is still little early attention to dispel the myths about vaccines, lack of trust in governments, and spread of misinformation and disinformation through social media before the distribution of vaccines.

Contemporary Globalization and Public Health

There are many approaches to study modern-day globalization and the processes that are changing the nature of human interactions and subsequent influences on health patterns and outcomes. In 2003, Kelley Lee[16] presented a conceptual multifactorial approach to study the direct and indirect impacts of globalization and health. This framework illustrates how the socio-cultural, political, economic, environmental, and technological spheres intersect across the spatial, temporal, and cognitive dimensions to fully show the interrelationship of globalization and public health. This approach moves beyond the narrower focus of how far and how fast globalization may influence public health and considers the cognitive dimension, offering a more critical analysis of Westernized influences on population mores, values, lifestyles, and behaviors. Furthermore, it proposes a growing unified consciousness influencing how we interact to what we eat, and where we live. Lee's premise was based upon the assumption that increased interaction leads toward greater connectedness and a convergence of such things as our values and behaviors, bringing both benefits and detriments to public health. For example, the desire for tropical fruits all year round or the accessibility to ethnic foods that one may have tasted at a restaurant or during an international excursion shows the increasing influence of globalization.

Microbes cross borders freely without a passport and can remain hidden from an unsuspecting traveler or within the traded goods, until it spreads. The reality is that with increased frequency, intensity, and convergence of people and goods, an infectious disease threat can emerge anywhere and go unnoticed until it strikes. In contemporary times, we know an epidemic in Madagascar could impact Mexico. The spread of diseases has been understood within a "political, legal, and commercial history of nationalism, colonialism, and internationalism..."[17]; therefore, history and geopolitics remain important. As mentioned earlier, Sholte's analysis of the deterritorialization or transplanetary connection of globalization can be applied to the wider public health issues. For example, importation of raspberries into the United States was doubling annually when cyclospora, a parasitic infection, hit the United States in 1996. The U.S. outbreak was blamed at first on strawberries from California, until further epidemiologic evidence traced it back to raspberries imported from Guatemala. While it took a few years to confirm the origin, Guatemalan Growers Association agreed to halt exporting raspberries. Many growers reduced their production over the years with economic losses,[18] and today most raspberries imported to the United States arrive from Mexico and Chile.

The role globalization has and will continue to play in the spread of infectious diseases reflects upon how we live, travel, and play. The growing ecotourism industry, offering unique travel opportunities to more remote regions in Latin America and the Caribbean with the promise of thrill-seeking activities, poses public health challenges. For example, leptospirosis, which is spread by exposure to urine or animals infected with the bacteria, also called mud fever, is the most widely spread zoonotic disease that is also underreported. This bacterial disease can cause a wide range of symptoms from headache, fever, chills, muscle aches, vomiting or diarrhea to no symptoms at all,[19] making it difficult to diagnose. It has become a more important disease to this region along with an increasing understanding about the spatial, temporal, and behavior dimensions. The highest prevalence is found in poor regions and among marginalized population, with ecotourism and water sports an important factor in travel-related diseases. The ecological changes related to human inference with deforestation, land erosion, or development projects such as dam construction to meet the needs of growing population are all important to land use and land change, disasters, and vectors of disease transmission.

Pappas et al. reported the highest rates of leptospirosis in the Caribbean and Central and South America, as well as Southeast Asia and Oceania regions with important environmental and social implications.[20] In Chapter 4 you will see how this zoonotic disease is also associated with natural disasters. There may be a panoply of reasons for the re-emergence of leptospirosis and regional environmental impact as well as travel and migration as important factors. A leptospirosis diagnosis has become more common with international travelers, even though there is underreporting due to lack of knowledge and diagnostic tests. Research conducted by Medhani Bandara et al.[21] shows a high prevalence in economically disadvantaged communities, including both poor urban centers lacking infrastructure for water and sewage and rural residents working in rice and sugar cane fields. Their research focused on the global spread of leptospirosis through travel and ecotourism with results showing that the trend for disease transmission has shifted to Latin America and the Caribbean islands as new locations for disease transmission were found among returning German travelers.

Rise of Noncommunicable Diseases and the Epidemiologic Transition

The study of infectious diseases associated with trade, travel, and tourism is not new. Focusing only on infectious diseases limits our understanding of the broader underlying factors contributing to good and poor population health outcomes. Also, it helps to explain the changing epidemiological patterns associated with noncommunicable diseases. Globalization is based upon liberal economic theories, with the assumption that more market competition produces better economic outcomes and consequently improving health outcomes. While health outcomes have improved, they have not improved equally within and across the Western Hemisphere.

To examine contemporary globalization and health, beyond the sole focus of infectious diseases, we also consider the expanding role of multinational corporations in industries such as the food and beverage, pharmaceutical, and tobacco. For example, the research on Peru and Bolivia showed a positive association of foreign direct investment with the prevalence of diet-related noncommunicable diseases.[22] Another example is the shift in tobacco consumption where more girls than boys are smoking in Argentina and Chile. The political economy of health is important to not only the study of diseases of poverty but also the rise in noncommunicable diseases in Latin America and the Caribbean. The marketing controversy continues about the role and responsibility of transnational corporations in protecting population health, unethical marketing practices, and future considerations of globalization and health support an analysis of the CDoH. This is significant since noncommunicable diseases are approximately 66% of the global burden of diseases in the Americas including all cancers, cardiovascular diseases, diabetes, strokes, and obesity. Additionally, there is a deep concern for co-morbidity risk of communicable and noncommunicable diseases.

Case Study 3.1

Nestlé Corporation's Unscrupulous Marketing Tactics

One of the first cases recognized for violating the codes of conduct by a transnational corporation was filed against the Nestlé Corporation. Criticisms began in the 1960s; however, it wasn't until 1981 that the WHO/UNICEF International Code of Marketing of Breast-Milk Substitutes was approved by the World Health Assembly. This was based upon a reasoning that Nestlé Corporation exercised unscrupulous marketing tactics to entice new mothers to use infant formula in Latin America as well as Africa and Asia. The promotion of infant formula as a substitute for breastfeeding, specifically in LMICs, provoked considerable concern throughout the international public health community.

This controversy erupted in Europe in 1974 after a pamphlet, The *Baby Killers*, avowed that infant formula provided less nutritional benefit than breastfeeding, thereby posing a health risk to infants.[23] Subsequently, consumer and activist groups participated in a well-organized and widespread boycott calling for Nestlé to change how they marketed baby formula. It was the 1977 boycott against Nestlé Corporation that triggered a global response. International corporations saw this as an attack on neoliberal free trade agreements, while critics maintained that it was a matter of health and safety associated with rising infant mortality rates. Opponents argued that the formula was provided to mothers, with free samples, while they were in the hospital. Then mothers with their newborns would return to homes without potable water (and use of surface water sources), no refrigeration, low literacy rates, and limited funds to purchase the formula. Families frequently had to use unclean water and leave unused portions of milk unrefrigerated, while mothers tried to stretch out the purchased milk by watering it down and reducing the nutritional value. This placed vulnerable infants at risk, with diarrhea and respiratory diseases contributing to rising infant mortality rates associated with this controversy. The call to boycott Nestlé products increased further through lawsuits and persistent public pressure. Ultimately, in 1984 Nestlé signed an agreement with the collaborative International Nestlé Boycott Committee (INBC) to terminate such practices in exchange for withdrawing boycotts against the corporation.

International Code of Marketing of Breast-Milk Substitutes

The purpose of the WHO/UNICEF's International Code of Marketing of Breast-Milk Substitutes adopted in May 1981 was to establish standards of ethical behavior, protect infant nutrition, and promote breastfeeding practices. In a 181-1 vote, the United States was the only country to vote against adopting the code to restrict marketing and promoting baby formula item. The Assistant Secretary of State remarked that the United States could not support the ban on advertising since it would "run counter to our constitutional guarantees for free speech and freedom of information."[24] One major contention was to stop the idealization of bottle feeding depicting ringlet blond hair rosy cheeked babies on their labels. Such standards called for restricting free samples to hospitals or health facilities; terminating the use of salespeople dressed as "milk nurses"; eliminating the coercive gifts to health workers; requiring labels to replace photos romanticizing the practice of formula use; including simple instructions on both breastfeeding and the risk of bottle feeding; presenting product information based on the scientific evidence; and lastly confirming that all products are of highest standard with consideration for the climate, temperature, and storage conditions of products.[25]

Baby Formula and Evidence of Risks in Low- and Middle-Income Countries

While there were other corporations engaging in similar practices, Nestlé Corporation was targeted since it represented 20% of all infant formula sales,[26] with 40% of the sales to LMICs.[27] One of the tactics used was sending salespeople dressed up as "milk nurses" into hospitals and clinics to glorify bottle feeding over breastfeeding. This provoked a counterattack by physicians, public health researchers, and activists alleging Nestlé was propagating immoral marketing practices, and at the same time encouraging countries to ban such advertisements by restricting the importation and distribution of infant formula to developing countries.[28] For example, in 1960, Chile's breastfeeding rates declined dramatically in eight years, while Mexico showed a decline in breastfeeding with the introduction of baby formula from 60% to 40% from 1960 to 1966, respectively.[29] A 1969–1970 study conducted in rural Chile found that three times more deaths were occurring among infants consuming formula before the age of three months as compared to those receiving only breastmilk.[30] In urban Brazil, from 1984 to 1985, another study showed how the protection of breastfeeding during the early months was statistically significant in preventing deaths from both diarrhea and respiratory infections.[31] Even with the early scientific evidence about the negative consequences in promoting bottle feeding over breast feeding to resource poor communities, there was a slow international response with transnational corporate power and increased trade not giving equal consideration to the protection of infant health. Powerful transnational actors have great influence on decision making, while public health's power may be subjugated by such corporate hegemony.

Nestlé Corporation Agreement during a New Neoliberal Economic Order

In 1984 Nestlé finally agreed to make adjustments and the boycott of nongovernmental organizations came to an end, becoming an important historical milestone. This took place during the new neoliberal economic order promoting free trade with limited restrictions, at the same time when resource poor countries were calling for greater regulations on unchecked multinational corporations. With the United States the only dissenter, it was the collective actions of governments, international organizations, civil society, faith-based institutions, and other transnational corporations that successfully brought this to fruition. Kathryn Sikkink captures this Nestlé infant formula controversy by examining the "theories of the formation and transformation of international regimes, which focus on behavior and expectations that converge around common set of principles, norms, rules, and procedures."[32] Her research provides a thorough analysis of the content on this issue, the context of different state and nonstate international actors, and the setting in which these actions take place.[33] This also offers an important contribution to the public health reality in the era of neoliberal trade structures.

Reflections From Latin America

I saw this in the 1980s in rural Latin America where women struggled to have clean water for baby formula, lived without electrical power or cold boxes to ensure the safety of consuming the leftover unrefrigerated formula, and were poorly informed about the dangers of diluting the milk. From Honduras to Colombia, I was no longer shocked after the first time I heard, "¿Está bien mezclar la fórmula con Coca-Cola?" (Is it ok to mix the formula with Coca-Cola?) Possibly this was fueled by a public health education campaign underway during this time to prevent infant and child deaths from diarrhea and dehydration. The promotion of a homemade oral rehydration solution, using an empty Coca-Cola liter bottle filled with water, a pinch of salt, and a scoop of sugar was a simple and effective way to reduce child deaths. The teaching of this practice was followed by a reminder, if it tastes saltier than tears throw it out and start again. This clear message offered a low literacy home-based approach to provide electrolytes and save lives. The ubiquitous Coca-Cola bottles may have seemed like good health education tool to use at the time.

The increasing access to both good and poor public health messaging reached its pinnacle for me while conducting field surveys with the Shipibo Indians along the Ucayali River in the central eastern portion of the Amazon in Pucallpa, Peru. It was 1983–1984 and the arrival of Western magazines showcased the new marketing strategies to help women lose weight and slim down. These glamorous flawless photos and advertisements were well placed to cajole readers to purchase products, suggesting that you too could look like just like these ad model women. Fortunately, such products were not available there at this time. Nevertheless, it did not stop confused women from reaching out to ask me if I thought by taking these products they would actually look like these pictures, e.g. blond hair and light skin young women. Inappropriate and just wrong! It was difficult to explain the misperceptions and the realities that undernutrition and insufficient micronutrients would be their priority. The idealization of such products continues as a poor display of the Westernized perceptions and related images of health. Sadly, this was similar to the assumption that buying Gerber food products would make your own infant look just like the rubicund baby displayed on the label. These events were all happening before the Internet reach of today.

The manufactured crisis of baby formula exemplified the new economic order that collided with public health. The disputes were not transpiring from government-to-government; rather, this dispute occurred between a powerful transnational corporation and governments with the wider engagement of civil society and nongovernmental organizations. Today we see such investor-government settlement disputes, a influence of the WTO, and continuing public health controversies that try to balance the benefits and detriments of globalization and public health.

Conclusion

The infant formula debate has been further complicated by the WHO's 1987 statement warning HIV+ mothers against breastfeeding. This was based upon the new evidence that the virus could be transmitted from mother-to-child through breastfeeding. With high rates of HIV/AIDS in the Americas, this issue became important to the furtherance of public health education. However, in 2010, the WHO presented new guidelines, with updated recommendations, based upon the wider accessibility

of antiretroviral drugs to treat pregnant mothers and prevent such transmission to their child. This also considered the significance of the underlying social determinants. According to a 2015 statement by Dr. Carissa
Etienne, Director of Pan American Sanitation Bureau (The Secretariat of
PAHO), mother-to-child transmission has seen a reduction by 50% since
2010, and such transmission was thereafter "considered eliminated as a
public health problem."[34]

A recent study on the infant formula debate revealed that infant mortality rates were 55% higher than the mean mortality rates used in the
sample households that depend upon surface drinking water, mothers
with less than primary education, and families living below poverty
levels.[35] This study illustrates that there are "significant infant mortality deaths from formula introduction concentrated in vulnerable
sub-populations,"[36] and consequently, this must take into account the
underlying social determinants as well as the CDoH. Once again, the
provision and sustainable access to safe water, education, and income remains the goal for better public health outcomes.

Today, the WHO recommends HIV+ mothers living in resource
poor regions of the world to continue to breastfeed, while for the United
States, the CDC recommends against it. In 2018, The Global Breastfeeding Initiative, consisting of more than 20 groups, stated that HIV+ mothers can breastfeed without the negative consequences as long as mothers
are taking antiretroviral medicine, since the risk of mother-to-child
transmission is extremely low.[37] Evidently, this controversy is ongoing.
Likewise, I wonder about the extent of influence transnational corporations will continue to have in this debate. While there is wide acceptance
of social determinants, further attention to the commercial determinants
of public health is essential.

Contemporary Trade and Public Health

The first multilateral trade agreement, the General Agreement on Trade and
Tariffs (GATT), was signed into law on January 1, 1948 and continued until it
was replaced by the WTO on January 1, 1995. The WTO created free trade
agreements, thereby reducing barriers and promoting the flow of exchanges
across borders. In the Americas, the North American Free Trade Agreement
(NAFTA) was established to enforce its own trade standards that fall outside
the WTO. The NAFTA allowed a country to refuse access to goods or services
based on scientific evidence; however, the burden fell upon the complaining
country, while under the WTO the responsibility falls upon the defending
country. As discussed in Chapter 2, the Commission of Social Determinants

of Health recognized that trade agreements and health equity must include the hazards of poor working conditions, substandard pay, exposures to unhealthy environment, or production of materials, which all could be a detriment to health. On December 10, 2019, the NAFTA was replaced with a new regional agreement between the United States, Mexico, and Canada (USMCA), which included a focus on the protection of workers, especially in Mexico. This went into effect on July 2, 2020, as the pandemic spread throughout the region.

The relationship of globalization to public health is closely associated with trade agreements and health policies. The role transnational actors play, especially multinational corporations, reveals both the positive and negative aspects of trade and public health outcomes such as access to knowledge, goods, and services, along with the circumstances of displacement, migration, and civil conflicts. The significance of globalization's indirect relationship may be unheeded in place of assessing the easier direct impacts on population health. The compression of globalization activities since the 1990s is observed through the rise in large corporation company ownership in a new economic order of trade liberalization. However, the increase in the privatization industrial growth did not necessarily consider how public health would fit into the dialogue. The idea of protectionism versus openness to free market and the role trade would play in reducing poverty and improve health created new opportunities and challenges. The early evidence of liberalized trade agreements was seen in the agricultural sector. The increased use of pesticides, fertilizers, as well as hormones and antibiotics in animals brought about a rapid transition in the availability and use of new foods, faster production of chickens, with improved technology and additives to extend the shelf life of foods.

Trade and Food Safety

As engagement in world trade increased, so did the concern for food safety and security. What became more apparent was that international food production complexes were controlled by a few big corporations where disease outbreak occurred. Consequently, more supervision was warranted. A joint Food and Agriculture Organization/WHO Codex Alimentarius Commission was established in 1963 and today has 188 Codex member countries and the European Union as a member organization collaborating to develop standards for food safety. What is important to recognize is that the WTO is the only organization governing the global trade, of which health and health-related trade is not necessarily a traditional concern in international trade policies. The WTO functions to provide technical assistance, administer, implement, and monitor trade agreements; it also serves to resolve disputes, while the WHO works to ensure such WTO agreements on trade do no harm public health. Under the WTO agreements, health protection is associated with such things as infectious disease control, food safety, tobacco, environment, access to drugs, health services, food security, nutrition, and biotechnology. The creation of the Sanitary and Phytosanitary Measures (SPS) agreements, which are international standards to achieve health objectives based upon good scientific evidence to protect humans, animals, and plants, allows governments to restrict trade in order to achieve such health objectives. Nevertheless, the WTO wording suggests appropriate level of SPS protection that would not minimize the negative trade effects.[38]

Trade, Foreign Direct Investment, and Nutritional Transition

The removal of trade barriers, competing transnational corporations, large foreign investments, along with deep pockets of advertising to promote obesogenic products marketed by the food and beverage industry has become a global public health problem The transition of diets, tastes, and health profiles from the '*burgerization*' *of* McDonalds to '*coca-colonization*' of coke products pushing the spread of eating habits from the North to the South and East to the West offers insights on diet, trade, and the nutritional transition. The globesity epidemic is no longer just a problem of rich countries, and has spread across Latin America and the Caribbean, presenting the paradox of both under- and over-nutrition co-existing.

This nutritional transition is also closely related to trade liberalization, foreign direct investment, and how free trade agreements have welcomed the arrival of foods high in fats, sugar, and sodium, adding flavoring, and extending the shelf life of packaged goods, After the NAFTA (1994), Mexico became the largest consumer of sugar-sweetened drinks in the world. A study assessing trade, foreign direct investment, and food consumption found a positive association of foreign direct investment with the prevalence of direct-related non-communicable diseases in middle-income countries. Researchers examined the free trade agreements in Peru in contrast to Bolivia, which had no such trade agreements, and found that such agreements did influence both the volume and type of foods and drinks available for purchase.[39]

I saw this recently. It was a typically hot breezy January 2018 morning when I awoke early from my hammock to hear the familiar sounds of young children, some as young as one year of age. I watched as they chomped down on cheesy crunchy-like snacks that stained their fingers as they licked the orange excess smacking their lips. These highly prized novelty treats arrive from Colombian or Panamanian transport boats. My residence, as I have traveled to Guna Yala, Panama over the many decades, overlooks the main dock where I can hear the chattering of people harmonize with the clicking sound of sandals along the aging cement pavement. This is often my alarm clock. This particular morning a Colombian trading boat arrived to purchase the plentiful coconuts from the island community and sell their products. The arrival of sugary sweet drinks, cookies, fatty-fried treats, and more is important to understand the nutritional transition associated with globalization.

I have spent many hours listening to wise Guna elders and chiefs. One of the most revered *sahila* (chief) was Gonzalo Salcedo, who was also a well-respected traditional healer, see Chapter 1. Gonzalo frankly expressed his concern about the youth consuming all the sugary items when fields of the sugar cane were growing right in front of their island community. He thought there was an outright laziness against harvesting the sugar cane for easy access and over-consumption of imported white sugar. He questioned, repeatedly, about the benefit of the processed and sugary foods and spoke out against the arrival of costly Westernized foods having a negative impact on the health of his beloved community. Gonzalo died in 2020, as have many of the elders with similar concerns about the changes in dietary habits. While less mobile and with in-creased hearing loss, he was never shy to express his opinion about Westernized influences on indigenous populations. In non-Western terms, he presented a prophetic analysis of the negative and positive outcomes of globalization and public health, which I must say offer profound insights beyond what many scholars can offer.

In Central America, nutrition associated with dietary patterns and free trade agreements with the United States has changed tariffs and non-tariff barriers, revealing how trade policy is correlated to food availability and food imports.[40] The increased consumption of processed foods is related to the wider access to such products in Latin American markets, with an increase from 15% in 1990 to 60% in 2000. In 2014, Mexico made two major regulatory changes by tax-ing unhealthy foods that were high in either one or more saturated fats, sugar, or sodium, and also placing a tax on sugar-sweetened beverages. What they found was a decline in purchase of taxed beverages with the greatest impact on low-income households. This study suggested wider implications of how taxa-tion can be used to promote behavior change.[41] Mexico has successfully taxed sugary beverages and lowered their consumption rates.

The demographic, epidemiologic, and health transitions evolved over time. The shift from hunter gatherers dying at a young age from infectious diseases, to subsistence farming and declining famines and pandemics allowed people to live longer. This was followed by the increased use of sugars, fats, caloric drinks, and processed foods, with a shift toward increasing communicable dis-eases, and a better pathway to healthier aging. The nutritional transition con-siders the shift of malnutrition from under to over nutrition, where historically the concern was undernutrition. Today malnutrition presents a different face. Latin American rural women have a higher prevalence of obesity than urban, but urban women may be catching up. The concern for energy imbalance associated with access to cheap cooking oils, increased consumption of empty calories from sugar and sugary soft drinks and highly processed foods, reduced physical activity, and changes in transportation recounts the story of globalization and public health.

Trade and Pharmaceuticals

Health protection becomes a costly battle when states engage in disputes over trade agreements. One of the greatest areas of trade disagreements has been waged against the pharmaceutical industry's use of trade-related intellectual property rights (TRIPS). The neoliberal economic paradigm pits the economic control against a public health counter argument to provide greater access to drugs, and especially lifesaving medicines. Weaker nation-states find it difficult to reject TRIPS if they want to participate and gain a greater share of the market.

The WTO created the compulsory license to produce lifesaving drugs with the caveat that they are manufactured only for use within the country. Under a clause of the TRIPS agreement, governments have the right to receive a compulsory license for limited purposes during a public health emergency, allowing them to use the intellectual property without gaining the permission from a pharmaceutical company that holds the drug patent. The height of this controversy occurred with HIV/AIDS, where Latin America and the Caribbean reported the second highest number of cases in the world behind the continent of Africa. Brazil, specifically, documented the second highest number of cases of HIV/AIDS globally in 1988, five years after the first case was diagnosed in the country. In 1996 highly active antiretroviral therapy (HAART) was developed using what has become known as a cocktail of different drugs that would keep HIV+ people alive. Sadly, the costs and access to these drugs were out of reach in LMICs. In 1996, however, Brazil became the first LMIC country to commit to and implement policies that would provide free access to HAART for HIV+ patients, thereby becoming a global model for increased access to lifesaving drugs.[42] In 2000, Brazil threatened to produce generic versions of HIV/AIDS drugs if the pharmaceutical industry would not reduce their costs significantly. The drug manufactured by Merck Pharmaceutical cost $1.60 for each pill, while in India it was less than 50 cents. In 2001, Brazil's Minister of Health, José Serra, authorized a Brazilian pharmaceutical company to produce the patented HIV/AIDS drug, Nelfinavir, which led to talks with other pharmaceutical companies agreeing to reduce the costs up to 60% for the cocktail of five different HIV/AIDS drugs. In 2007 Brazil was one of the first countries to approve a compulsory license for a generic form of HIV/AIDS drug, Efavirenz. A variety of stakeholders from the then Minister of Health, José Gomes Temporão, to civil society social movements motivated action to bring the cost down through this compulsory licensing agreement. Brazil became the model for LMIC in response to HIV/AIDS scaling up programs for essential medicines making them more accessible. Since 2013, Brazil has provided antiretroviral treatment free for all HIV+ people.

Developing a new drug or therapeutic requires large infusion of capital, time, and expertise from research to marketing. It can take a decade or more to develop a new drug, so protecting trademark patents for up to 20 years – before it can go off label as a generic – may seem like a justified practice. Unless, of course, the drug is so costly that it is prohibitive for most people to have access to the lifesaving drugs. HIV/AIDS advocacy to activism made the access to life-saving drugs a human right and galvanized a movement that brought a human face to trade and health.

Trade, Foreign Direct Investment and Tobacco

There is a long history of trade and tobacco in the Americas. The Spanish supported it in the Dominican Republic, Portuguese in Brazil, and British in the United States; however, it wasn't until the 1900s that tobacco became a big business industry. Tobacco use contributes to noncommunicable diseases and premature deaths, is a drain on the health care system, and disproportionately impacts the poor today. Disturbingly tobacco is legally traded, yet, when used as directed kills.

Cancer is one of the main causes of adult death in Latin America and the Caribbean,[43] of which lung cancer is increasing among males in Argentina, Chile, and Cuba. Even with a decline in smoking rates in Brazil and Mexico, women are using tobacco in increasing rates. This is a concern since the feminization of tobacco – using targeted marketing strategies – shows 13–14-year old boys and girls in Brazil, Colombia, and Uruguay reporting equal smoking rates, with increased rates among girls in Argentina and Chile. Noteworthy is the rise in smokeless tobacco products.

In 2003 the WHO adopted its first global public health treaty, the Framework Convention on Tobacco Control (FCTC). The FCTC is a binding agreement for WHO member states to address both the demand and supply of tobacco products and consider the public health impacts. Nevertheless, trade, sale, marketing, and consumption of tobacco products remains a major global public health challenge with increasing rates in LMIC.

Economic consumption theory supports how LMIC nations became vulnerable to trade liberalization with increased tobacco use. Countries compete for transnational tobacco corporations to invest in their country, bringing tax benefits and employment opportunities. Big tobacco is efficient in generating the demand for products by getting governments to reduce prices and increase demand. Consequently, increased trade and competition will reduce prices, making tobacco products more accessible and with increased advertising, they can reach new markets.

The decline of tobacco consumption in higher income countries pushed the tobacco industry toward LMICs. TRIPS gave corporations the right to sue countries for failure to adhere to the agreed regulations under the WTO.

The landmark case of Uruguay is one of the best examples to show how disputes have transitioned from government-to-government to investor disputes against governments, while Uruguay was actively engaged in anti-smoking strategies.[44] In 2010 Philip Morris International (PMI), known for its most famous tobacco product, Marlboro, sued the government of Uruguay when the country placed public health restrictions to protect their population from harmful effects of tobacco. In 2009, Uruguay implemented a law that required all cigarette packaging to contain health warnings and graphic images. PMI argued that since a pre-existing bilateral treaty between Uruguay and Switzerland (the home based for PMI) continued, such restrictions were in violation of the agreement and damaged their reputation. The WTO International Centre for Settlement of Investment Disputes ruled against PMI for $7 million in 2016. It took six years for Uruguay to win the suit brought against them by PMI.[45] Uruguay's ability to fight this in court was made possible through the assistance of American billionaire philanthropist Michael Bloomberg Foundation, who also provided the money to challenge the tobacco giant. This has been referred to as a David win over Goliath and the triumph of public health over big business profits. In 2016 the Michael Bloomberg Foundation was appointed Global Ambassador for Noncommunicable Diseases and committed $350 million to reduce tobacco use.

Concluding Remarks

I began this chapter by sharing my astonishment in witnessing barges piled high with cases of Coca-Cola motoring toward more remote communities along the Magdalena River in Colombia. Many decades later, the promotion of unhealthy products is no less disconcerting, while globalization continues to offer both benefits and detriments to public health. Recognizing the social determinants of health and CDoH corroborates why the different stakeholders and perspectives are fundamental to this discussion.

The challenge is to develop a logical approach to trade that includes public health protection. Many researchers call for more public health investigation in this area. Walls, Baker, and Smith suggest using methods adapted from political science and management studies to improve upon negotiations, conflict, and the necessary decision-making strategies.[46] Promoting a more robust research platform across disciplines and sectors within a government partnership could provide a better way to understand the direct and indirect impacts of trade activities, trade agreements, foreign direct investments, and public health consequences. Friel et al. suggests that a health impact analysis considers human rights assessment.[47] This will require greater cooperation across the many stakeholders and their competing interests, in order to attain policy coherence and protect the rights and well-being of peoples. Furthermore, it underscores why diplomacy is another essential component in the study and practice of public health, which will be discussed in Chapter 5.

Notes

1 Refer to Chapter 2, "Development and Public Health," for more information.
2 Gerald Hastings, "Why Corporate Power Is a Public Health Priority," *British Medical Journal (BMJ)* 345 (2012): e5124.
3 John S. Millar, "The Corporate Determinants of Health: How Big Business Affects Our Health, and the Need for Government Action," *Canadian Journal of Public Health* 104, (2013): e327–329.
4 Ibid.
5 Iona Kickbush, Luke Allen, and Christian Franz, "Commercial Determinants of Health," *The Lancet* 4 (2016): 395–396.
6 Melissa Mailon et al., "The Architecture of the State Was Misinformed in Favour of the Interests of Companies: Corporate Political Activity of the Food Industry in Colombia," *Globalization and Health* 16, no. 97 (2020), doi:10.1186/s12992-020-00631-x.
7 Harold Jacobson, *Networks of Interdependence: International Organizations and Global Political System* (New York: Knopf, 1979), 33.
8 Giovanni Berlinguer, "The Interchange of Disease and Health between the Old and New Worlds," *American Journal of Public Health* 82 (1992): 1407–1413.
9 Ibid.
10 See Michael D. Martin et al., "Genomic Characterization of a South American *Phytophthora* Hybrid Mandates Reassessment of the Geographic Origins of *Phytophthora infestans*," *Molecular Biology and Evolution* 33, no. 2 (2016): 478–491, doi:10.1093/molbev/msv241; and Joseph Caspermeyer, "The South American Origins and Spread of the Irish Potato Famine Pathogen," *Molecular Biology and Evolution* 33, no. 3 (2016): 862, doi:10.1093/molbev/msv278.
11 Ulysses B. Panisett, *International Health Statecraft: Foreign Policy and Public Health in Peru's Cholera's Epidemic* (Lanham, MD: Rowan & Littlefield, 2000).
12 World Health Organization, Global Task Force on Cholera Control, *Cholera Unveiled* (Geneva: WHO, 2003), 4. http://whqlibdoc.who.int/hq/2003/WHO_CDS_CPE_ZFK_2003.3.pdf.
13 Centers for Disease Control and Prevention, "The History of Smallpox," accessed June 11, 2020, https://www.cdc.gov/smallpox/history/history.html.
14 Donald G. McNeil, Jr., "Wary of Attack with Smallpox, U.S. Buys up a Costly Drug," *The New York Times*, March 12, 2013, https://www.nytimes.com/2013/03/13/health/us-stockpiles-smallpox-drug-in-case-of-bioterror-attack.html.
15 Adriana Guzman-Holtz et al., "Barrier to Vaccination in Latin America: A Systematic Literature Review," *Vaccine* 38, no. 3 (2020): 470–481.
16 Kelley Lee, *Globalization and Health: An Introduction*, Global Issues Series (New York: Palgrave Macmillan, 2003).
17 Alison Bashford, "The Age of Universal Contagion: History, Disease and Globalization," in *Medicine at the Border: Disease, Globalization and Security, 1850 to Present*, ed. Alison Bashford (London: Palgrave Macmillan, 2007), 1–14.
18 Dan Flynn, "Last Big Cyclopora Outbreak Was Traced to Guatemalan Raspberries," *Food Safety News*, July 19, 2013, https://www.foodsafetynews.com/2013/07/last-big-cyclospora-outbreak-was-traced-to-guatemalan-raspberries/.
19 See Centers for Disease Control and Prevention on Leptospirosis for Further Information: https://www.cdc.gov/leptospirosis/index.html.

20 Georgios G. Pappas, et al. "The globalization of leptospirosis: worldwide incidence trends." *Int J Infect Dis 12.* no 4 (2008): 351–357

21 Medhani Bandara et al., "Globalization of Leptospirosis through Travel and Migration," *Globalization and Health* 10, no. 61 (2014). doi:10.1186/s12992-014-0061-0.

22 Philip Baker et al., "Trade and Investment Liberalization, Food Systems Change and Highly Processed Food Consumption: A Natural Experiment Contrasting the Soft-Drink Markets of Peru and Bolivia," *Globalization and Health* 12 (2016), doi:10.1186/s12992-016-0161-0.

23 The British Nongovernmental Organization, War on Want, published a booklet written by Mike Muller in March 1974: *The Baby Killers: A War on Want Investigation into the Promotion and Sale of Powdered Baby Milk in Developing Countries,* http://archive.babymilkaction.org/pdfs/babykiller.pdf.

24 Stephen Solomon, "Controversy over Infant Formula", *The New York Times,* December 6, 1981, https://www.nytimes.com/1981/12/06/magazine/the-controversy-over-infant-formula.html.

25 Naomi Baumslag and Dia L Michels, *Milk, Money and Madness: Culture and Politics of Breastfeeding* (Westwood, CT: Greenwood Publishing, 1995).

26 Ibid.

27 S. Prakash Sethi, *Multinational Corporations and the Impact of Public Advocacy on Corporate Strategy: Nestlé and the Infant Formula Controversy* (Norwell, MA: Kluwer Academic Publishers, 1994).

28 Ibid.

29 Jesse K Anttilla-Hughes et al., *Mortality from Nestlé's Marketing of Infant Formula in Low and Middle-Income Countries* (Working Paper) (Cambridge, MA: National Bureau of Economic Research, 2018), 16.

30 Stephen J. Plank and Maria Lucila Milanesi, "Infant Feeding and Infant Mortality in Rural Chile," *Bulletin of the World Health Organization* 48 (1973): 203–210.

31 Cesar G. Victora et al., "Evidence for Protection by Breast-Feeding against Infant Deaths from Infectious Diseases in Brazil," *The Lancet* 2, no. 8554 (1987): 319–322, doi:10.1016/s0140-6736(87)90902-0.

32 Kathryn Sikkink, "Codes of Conduct for Transnational Corporations: The Case Study of WHO/UNICEF Code," *International Organization* 40, no. 4 (1986): 816.

33 Ibid.

34 Pan American Health Organization, *Elimination of Mother-to-Child Transmission of HIV and Syphilis in the Americas. Update 2015* (Washington, DC: PAHO, 2015).

35 Jesse K. Anttilla-Hughes et al., *Mortality from Nestlé's Marketing of Infant Formula in Low and Middle-Income Countries* (Working Paper) (Cambridge, MA: National Bureau of Economic Research, 2018).

36 Ibid, 7.

37 World Health Organization and United Nations Children's Fund, *Advocacy Brief: Breastfeeding and HIV: Global Breastfeeding Collective* (Geneva: World Health Organization, 2019).

38 See Sharon Friel, Libby Hattersley, and Ruth Townsend, "Trade Policy and Public Health," *Annual Review of Public Health* 36 (2015): 325–344, and Helen Walls, Phillip Baker, and Richard Smith, "Moving Toward Policy Coherence in Trade and Health," *Journal of Public Health Policy* 36, no. 4 (2015): 491–501.

39 Philip Baker et al., "Trade and Investment Liberalization, Food Systems Change and Highly Processed Food Consumption: A Natural Experiment Contrasting the Soft-Drink Markets of Peru and Bolivia," *Globalization and Health* 12 (2016), doi:10.1186/s12992-016-0161-0.

40 Anne Marie Thow and Corinna Hawkes, "The Implications of Trade Liberalization for Diet and Health: A Case Study from Central America," *Globalization and Health* 5, no. 5 (2009), doi:10.1186/1744-8603-5-5.

41 M. Arantxa Colchreo et al., "In Mexico, Evidence of Sustained Consumer Response Two Years after Implementing a Sugar-Sweetened Beverage Tax," *Health Affairs* 36, no. 3 (March 2017), doi:10.1377/hlthaff.2016.1231.
42 Amy S Nunn et al., "Evolution of Antiretroviral Drug Costs in Brazil in the Context of Free and Universal Access to AIDS Treatment," *PLOS* (2007), doi:10.1371/journal.pmed.0040305.
43 Paul E. Goss et al., "Planning Cancer Control in Latin America and the Caribbean," *The Lancet: Oncology* 14, no. 5 (2013), doi:10.1016/S1470-2045(13)70048-2. This Commission included 72 investigators in 12 countries discussing obstacles in response to rising rates of cancer within and across the region.
44 Eduardo Bianco, Beatriz Champagne, and Joaquin Barnoya, "The Tobacco Epidemic in Latin America and the Caribbean: A Snapshot," *Prevention and Control* 1, no. 4 (2005): 311–317.
45 Eric Crosbie, Patricia Sosa, and Stanton A Glantz, "Defending Strong Tobacco Packaging and Labelling Regulations in Uruguay: Transnational Tobacco Network versus Philip Morris International," *British Medical Journal (BMJ)* 27 (2018): 185–193.
46 Helen Walls, Phillip Baker, and Richard Smith, "Moving Toward Policy Coherence in Trade and Health," *Journal of Public Health Policy* 36, no. 4 (2015): 491–501.
47 Sharon Friel, Libby Hattersley, and Ruth Townsend, "Trade Policy and Public Health," *Annual Review of Public Health* 36 (2015): 325–344.

Bibliography – Selected Books

de Salazar, Ligia Malagón and Lugan Villar, Roberto Carlos, eds., *Globalization and Health Inequities in Latin America*. New York City: Springer International Publishing, 2019.

Fidler, David P. *SARS, Governance and the Globalization of Disease*. New York: Palgrave Macmillan, 2004.

Fort, Meredith, Mercer, Mary Anne and Gish, Oscar, eds. *Sickness and Wealth- The Corporate Assault on Global Health*. Cambridge: South End Press, 2004.

Gilpin, Robert. *The Political Economy of International Relations*. Princeton, NJ: Princeton University Press, 1978.

Jacobson, Harold. *Networks of Interdependence: International Organizations and Global Political System*. New York: Knopf, 1979.

Kawachi, Ichiro and Wamala, Sarah, eds. *Globalization and Health*. Oxford: Oxford University Press, 2007.

Lee, Kelley. *Globalization and Health: An Introduction*. New York: Palgrave Macmillan, 2003.

Lee, Kelley, Buse, Kent, and Fustukian, Suzanne, eds. *Health Policy in a Globalising World*. Cambridge: Cambridge University Press, 2002.

McNeill, William H. *Plagues and Peoples*. New York: Anchor Books, Division of Random House, 1976 (1998 edition).

McNeill, John Robert. *Mosquito Empires: Ecology and War in the Grater Caribbean, 1620–1914, New Approaches to the Americas*. Cambridge: Cambridge University Press, 2010.

Strange, Susan. *States and Markets*. London: Bloomsbury Academic, 1988.

Vineis, Paolo. *Health without Borders- Epidemics in the Era of Globalization*. Cham: Springer International Publishing, 2017.

Youde, Jeremy. *Globalization and Health*. Lanham, MD: Rowman and Littlefield, 2020.

4

DISASTERS, CLIMATE CRISIS, AND PUBLIC HEALTH

Latin America and the Caribbean is the second most at risk region in the world to disasters. According to the United Nations Office for the Coordination of Humanitarian Affairs (OCHA), from 2000 to 2019 floods, hurricanes, earthquakes, landslides, volcanic eruptions, wildfires, droughts, and extreme temperatures have impacted 152 million people in the region. These events present significant public health and economic challenges that disproportionately impact the poor and indigenous populations. A major concern moving forward is that the frequency and intensity of disasters and climate crisis reveal a growing threat to the most vulnerable populations from highland to coastal communities throughout the region.

In 2017, the Pan American Health Organization (PAHO) asked countries to prioritize their major issues and challenges associated with health and climate change. Eighteen countries participated, including 15 member states and 3 territories in the region. The PAHO reported 11 issues ranked as extremely important or important with vector-borne diseases followed by weather and emergencies, food security and safety, and water-borne diseases as the top priorities for the Ministry of Health (MOH).[1] Throughout the region, the crossroads of disasters, climate change, and public health are a major concern now and for the future.

The prediction that climate change and droughts would arrive faster and become more intense especially in the Caribbean[2] was realized in 2015 when one of the worst droughts hit Central America and the Caribbean, followed by an extended dry season in the southern part of the Amazon, Brazil. Multiple storms, flooding, and devastating hurricanes are pummeling the Caribbean and upending the lives of thousands of people, damaging the ecology and destroying already fragile infrastructure and economies. This continues with a worldwide

DOI: 10.4324/9781003007401-5

alarm about the out of control wildfires in Brazil's Amazon rainforest, which began in 2019 and continue to burn a year later.

More silent than the roaring storms or scorching fires are the devasting droughts affecting the greatest number of people in Central America where crop losses have been reported as high as 50–75%. These unstable weather patterns from flooding to long periods of drought have impacted 2.2 million people in El Salvador, Guatemala, Honduras, and Nicaragua. This Northern Triangle of Central America, known as the Dry Corridor, extends from Southern Mexico to Panama with droughts, tropical storms, and consequent landslides, displacing many from their homes, especially residents in rural communities. The World Food Program (WFP) reported the damaging blow to maize and bean crops where farmers have confronted the worst dry cropping seasons in decades. The WFP forecasts a 60–80% probability that such extreme weather-related events will continue, creating migration as climate-induced displacements of communities' struggle to relocate. I have observed this growing alarm in Panama among the Guna Indians where sea level rise and intensity of rains and storms, even during the expected dry season, are threatening their livelihoods in the low-level islands they call home. In June 2019 discussions with elder leaders, all claim they have never seen anything quite like the recent intensity of rains, flooding, or heat waves. In January 2020, I was unable to travel from Panama City to the islands due to the rough seas that were declared as too dangerous for boat transport.

Naturally occurring climatic events related to the El Nino–Southern Oscillation (ENSO) cycle play another important role in public health in Latin America where populations are particularly vulnerable to natural disasters. The ENSO is a key contributor to climate variability with the most intensity found in the tropics. The ENSO measures the changing temperature between the ocean and atmosphere in the Equatorial Pacific identifying the fluctuation between the warm phase, El Niño, and the cool phase, La Niña. Research has shown that the ENSO effects many health determinants associated with the ecosystem and destruction to the public health infrastructure. Specific health outcomes associated with vector-borne and water-borne diseases have been documented with El Niño, and malaria in South America, and dengue in Central and South America. A warming climate may further contribute to both the intensity and frequency of El Niño in Latin America and the Caribbean as extreme rainfall and flooding in Caribbean while droughts may occur along the Pacific coastal states.

The cascading effect of disasters, climate, food insecurity, malnutrition, displacement, infectious diseases, and migration portrays a gloomy picture for public health, safety, and security of peoples. As the world confronts the greatest public health disaster in more than a century, the COVID-19 is a bleak reminder that disasters disrupt lives and economies beyond the short-term impact. A discussion on how this pandemic has impacted Latin America and the

Caribbean appears to seamlessly fit into this chapter. However, I have chosen to discuss the COVID-19 event as part of the concluding chapter. There I will provide a brief analysis about this pandemic and the interconnectedness to national and international development, globalization, disasters, diplomacy, and security, which will tie each chapter to one another in this book.

Brief History of Disasters in the Region

Historians appear to have neglected the study of natural disasters until more recent times.[3] What we do know throughout history is that weather- and geological-related disasters have caused far-reaching harm to people, the environment, and the economy.[4]

Flooding throughout history has been the cause of earlier famine and high death tolls. From 1312 to 1322, flooding caused famine throughout Northern Europe. While data are not available on the number of deaths, historian William Chester Jordan writes that up to 33% of the population died from diseases and hunger. His analysis was based upon reports maintained in monasteries, along with agricultural and meteorological documents that revealed fluctuating droughts, flooding, and cold winters, where he proposed that the "Great Famine" was associated with the interaction of weather changes coupled with social, economic, political instability, environmental, and poor health outcomes of diseases.[5] Fernand Braudel in *La Méditerranée et le Monde Méditerranéen à* (*The Mediterranean and Mediterranean World in the Age of Philip II*) (1949) discussed how the frequency of flooding contributed to such famines, where he also recognized the importance of the role humans played. Such behaviors associated with disasters, wars, famines, diseases, and other chaotic events show how cultural and societal changes take place when calamities such as natural disasters strike, suggesting that such events will disrupt and transform societies and institutions.[6] Schwartz uses these works to examine the history of disasters in the Caribbean within a broader context of the social and political factors, environment challenges, and human influences.[7] Therefore, applying multidimensional and multifactorial approaches offer the broader historical to current day understanding of the intersection of disasters and climate crisis with sociocultural, political, economic, environmental, and technological determinants.

In 1780, a hurricane in the Caribbean struck Martinique, St. Eustatius, and Barbados killing 80,000 people.[8] In 1812, a major earthquake struck Venezuela devastating Caracas and mobilizing a collective international response. A volcanic eruption of Mt. Pelée Martinique and St. Vincent in 1902 killed more than 30,000 people. Floods in Mexico, earthquakes in Chile and Nicaragua, and a significant storm in Dominican Republic all caused major destruction from the early to mid-1900s. Conceivably, the idea of disaster mitigation may have been established earlier in the Americas with the earthquake resilient architecture designed by the Incas in South America along with the Spanish

Colonial architecture.[9] We can look back in history to the biblical story of Noah's Ark, which many believe was inspired by the great floods of Mesopotamian and the Epic of Gilgamesh in which a number of Sumerian cities were wiped out. It could be argued that this supported the early warning message to prepare and mitigate against the Great Flood and provides another indication that the knowledge of mitigating disasters is not really a new occurrence.

Nevertheless, it was the Great Fire in London in 1666 that destroyed almost one-third of the city leaving thousands homeless and a damaged economy, which appears to be the first major disaster motivating specific actions for more training and improved strategies to reduce the loss of lives. It wasn't until 1859, with the founding of the International Federation of Red Cross (IFRC), that such organized humanitarian actions were implemented. It was Henry Dunant's efforts at the bloody battle in Solferino, Italy (June 24, 1859) where an estimated 40,000 men were left to die on the battlefield which shaped the IFRC.

Was saving lives on the battlefield the foundation upon which current day disaster management is based upon? I think not. Disaster management is more closely aligned with the fire service's controlling of wildfires where they established the incident command system to ensure effective and efficient response to emergency events, while protecting the health and safety of first responders. This is built into the training from local to global levels. We will see how disaster management has evolved and where gaps still remain, with examples from Latin America and the Caribbean.

Rise in Disaster Organizations in the Region

In 1976 the PAHO created the Emergency Preparedness Relief Coordination Program to address disasters and health emergencies in the region. Since the 1980s Latin America and the Caribbean has focused its attention on disaster management. It was the September 19, 1985 earthquake in Mexico and November 13, 1985 Nevado del Ruiz volcano eruption in Colombia that further spirited regional coordination to promote disaster mitigation efforts. In 1988 the *Centro de Coordinación para la Prevención de los Desastres Naturales en América Central* (CEPREDENAC), Coordination Center for the Prevention of Natural Disaster Prevention in Central America was soon followed by the Caribbean Disaster Emergency Response Agency (CDERA). CDERA was first created in 1991 as a regional response agency and ultimately became a more vigorous disaster management system under the Caribbean Community. *Red de Estudios Sociales en Prevención de Desastres en América (LA RED)*, Network of Social Studies on the Prevention of Disasters in Latin America, was formalized in Costa Rica in 1992 and became one of the earliest public-private partnerships for disaster risk reduction in the region with members from Brazil, Canada, Colombia, Costa Rica, Ecuador, Mexico, and Peru. Their important contribution shifted attention from perception of the concept of natural disaster to include the social construct of disasters. The demand for improved regional disaster information led to the 1997 *Centro Regional Información de Desastres*, to both disseminate and promote better information about disaster management throughout the region. The *Latino Americana de Centros de Informacìon en Gestìòn del Riesgo de Desatsre*s (Latin American Network for Disasters and Health Information), in collaboration with the PAHO, formed the Central American Network after Hurricane Mitch in 1998. Their purpose was to improve the sharing of health information in the poorest countries such as Honduras and Nicaragua that were severely impacted by Hurricane Mitch. The Comité Andino para la Prevención y Atención de Desastres (CAPRADE) Andean Committee for Disaster Prevention and Assistance was formed in 2002. The PAHO works closely with these regional groups. This is not meant to be a complete list. Rather, it shows the sub-regional focus on coordination, cooperation, and sustainable collaborative efforts for regional disaster management across the different catastrophes in Latin America and Caribbean over the past 40 years.

Classifying Disasters

Historically, disasters have been classified as natural, human-generated (man-made), and human-induced, or human conceived events. Now, we know that naturally occurring and human factors have become more important to how and at what level human behaviors contribute to the outcomes of natural disasters. Rigid classifications are not always useful. Natural disasters can be termed as geological- or weather-related such as tropical storms or hurricanes, earthquakes, volcanos, mudslides, floods, or droughts. A natural disaster can be a sudden impact or slow onset events associated with environmental degradation, droughts, deforestation, pests, and vermin destroying crops that can be influenced by anthropogenic factors. This is where public health has played an active role in studying ways to prevent, mitigate, prepare, and respond.

Beyond natural disasters are human-induced or human-generated events that can be unintentional or intentional events. These events have wide-reaching public health implications such as industrial or technological failures causing pollution, chemical, or radiation exposures, the deforestation and material shortages related to food, water, and the economy, and the elevated importance of the anthropogenic factors of carbon emissions contributing to climate change. A last major classification is often referred to as human conceived events such as the heinous crimes of ethnic cleansing, genocide, terrorist, or torturous acts. While important to global and regional population health, this will not be covered here.

Governments, multilateral institutions, and global to regional organizations classify emergency events based upon different priorities. Some use deaths, injuries, illnesses, while others apply economic costs, or frequency and intensity of events, and still others focus on how many people have been displaced during and after a specific incident. The health sector draws its attention to epidemiologic evidence, public health indicators, and access to infrastructure; the economic sector focuses on costs and losses of infrastructure and commerce; scientists and modelers focus on frequency and intensity with forecasting predictability and likelihood of future events, and humanitarian and human rights groups focus on the displacement and protection of the most vulnerable. All are crucial measures of disasters and population welfare and underscore the complexity of the issues, perspectives, actors, and methodologies applied to respond.

Disaster Risks

Understanding the overall risk of a disaster is associated with both the hazards and vulnerabilities of the population. Recognizing the likelihood of an event's impact requires having information about the hazards, which is based upon the history, underlying causes, frequency, and intensity of previous events. Also, identifying the most vulnerable populations and their potential public health impacts are part of risk-based analysis. According to the United Nations Development Program, vulnerability is "determined by physical, social, economic, and environmental factors or process, which increase susceptibility to the impact of hazard."[10]

In the Western Hemisphere hurricanes are the most frequent with more people affected and fewer deaths. These are based on the Saffir/Simpson Scale Categories I-IV measuring the wind speed and storm surge. The impact of wind, rain, and water surges threatens infrastructure and challenges governments to develop better policies that help mitigate and make the population more resilient to the impact of a disaster. Earthquakes cause the greatest death toll with huge economic costs. Therefore, improved policies, regulations, and enforcements are necessary to protect at-risk populations before, during, and after an earthquake. This includes such things as appropriate construction materials, location of homes and buildings, and sensible land use as part of the disaster prevention, mitigation, and preparedness to build community resilience. We know regulations are not equally implemented within and across the region. This was observed in the earthquake mitigation and resiliency strategies used in Chile and not in Haiti in 2010.

There is a growing field of research on climate change, the most at-risk or vulnerable populations, and the best practices to mitigate and promote resiliency at local community levels. The problem is putting the research into practice. As with other rigorous science-based public health protection the translation to evidence-based policies has not kept pace. The 2018 Global Risk Report found that climate and technology posed the greatest risk with Central America as one of the top hotspots. The World Economic Forum Global Risks Perception

Survey 2017–2018 reported that extreme weather and natural disasters, failures of climate mitigation and adaptation, and water crisis are expected to have the greatest impact over the next decade. The Global Risk Outlook for 2019 ranked the top three events likely to occur from the extreme weather events, followed by climate change mitigation and adaptation, and natural disasters.[11] The resounding reality of anticipated disasters and fear will co-exist as the call for more investments in prevention, mitigation, preparedness, and resiliency faces financial obstacles and limited political will to ensure implementation.

Disaster Management

Disasters present numerous challenges for population health, safety, and security; therefore, preventing such deleterious effects is an integral part of disaster management today. The cyclical process of disaster management starts from prevention, mitigation, preparedness, response, with the capacity to build resilience before the next event. This takes place while multiple emergency events compete for attention and economic resources to put the necessary steps into place, knowing that the different state and non-state actors within the region will cooperate or collide to prioritize their objectives. This also considers a relationship to the necessary actions taken during the different phases of a disaster. Prevention and mitigation strategies must begin well before a disaster strikes, and where the emergency response from search and rescue to recovery can demonstrate how communities are well prepared and more resilient to reduce loss of lives. This is followed by the post-event phase from short- to long-term rebuilding and advancing the lessons learned along the way. When I think about driving the attention to prevention and not the response, it reminds me of something I read decades ago by Kenneth Waltz, *Man, the State and War* (1959). "Asking who won a war, someone has said, is like asking who won the San Francisco earthquake. That in wars there is no victory but only varying degrees of defeat." In disasters there is only varying degrees of suffering.

Disaster Management Cycle: Examples from Latin America and the Caribbean

The development of Early Warning Systems (EWS) is an important tool to mitigate the loss of lives. After the 1985 earthquake where Mexico City experienced unprecedented deaths and damage even though the epicenter was not near the city, the government invested in early warnings for their most vulnerable areas. Significant contributions in technology and seismological studies have been beneficial to identifying the gaps in public policies and protocols for the dissemination of alerts. Social scientists recognized this as an essential element of the EWS from inception, highlighting the importance of bridging science with public policies.[12] Poor communication strategies were also identified as a reason why people did not leave when the volcán *Tungurahua* (throat of fire in Quechua) erupted in Ecuador in 2006. Tungurahua is one of the most active volcanoes in South America, with population risks from ash explosions, pyroclastic and lava flows, and displacement. Researchers, in collaboration with communities, designed better communication tools with appropriate language, engaging local residents in the monitoring and reporting information, and gaining the trust of populations to build a more resilient approach and reduce risks.[13]

We have seen the benefit of earthquake resiliency programs. In Haiti, a 7.0 magnitude earthquake hit 16 miles from the Capital city Port-au-Prince on Tuesday, January 12, 2010 at 4:53 pm, bringing about more than 200,000 deaths. While on Saturday, February 27, 2010 at 3:30 pm, an 8.8 earthquake struck 200 miles from Santiago, Chile, causing 300 deaths. With growing populations and growing demand for more buildings, Chile invested in earthquake resistant buildings, using engineering science coupled with enforcing building codes to protect livelihoods. Many lives were saved in Chile while the devastating toll in Haiti was ruinous.[14]

We know disasters disproportionately impact the poor from local to global levels. The consequence of Hurricane Katrina that made landfall as a Category 3 during the early morning hours of August 23, 2005 in New Orleans, Louisiana, was an unambiguous reminder. The intensity and frequency of hurricane devastation across small states in the Caribbean expose the reality of a societal fracture where a risk-based analysis must consider the hazards and vulnerability of populations, including the issues of environmental injustice, discrimination, and inequalities that place marginalized populations at even a higher risk during a disaster. Hurricane Dorian thrashed the Bahamas as a Category 5, striking Abaco Islands on September 1, 2019. This caused massive destruction and flooding in the northernmost islands, becoming the strongest hurricane recorded in the Atlantic Ocean and deemed the worst natural disaster to ever hit the country. The death toll is still unknown since missing people have been removed from the death toll list, according to the former Minister of Health Dr. Duane Sands, stating, "the country so badly botched its record keeping on Hurricane Dorian's missing victims that today it cannot say with certainty how many people actually died in the horrific storm."[15] An estimate $7 billion in damage, with an unequal toll it took on both the poor Bahamian residents and Bahamian Haitian immigrants, shows the blatant inequities seen in the aftermath of disasters. While the dominant, albeit important, discussion remains on the role of climate change and increasing intensity of hurricanes, we cannot overlook the structural determinants that have its roots in poverty and uneven development, class, colonization, and fundamental human rights of people. Von Meding et al. reminds us that decision-makers must include such social inequities as part of the rebuilding and reconstruction plans.[16]

Throughout history we have seen how the haste to rebuild after a disaster, with expectations to rush back to normal, is never an acceptable path when the structural determinants are not fully integrated into both the reconstruction of building and human lives. I've seen numerous times, whether it is an earthquake, landslide, flood, or hurricane, people returning to the same lands to rebuild with no support or policies in place to protect population from the next event.

Climate, Disasters, and Infectious Diseases

Temperature, humidity, and weather patterns influence the spread of infectious diseases as does the contributing factor of the intensity and frequency of disasters. An estimated 200 thousand deaths each year in the low- and middle-income countries (LMICs) will come from climate-related changes. Diarrhea, malnutrition, and vector-borne diseases are some key climate-sensitive health concerns that have the greatest toll on young children. Establishing better policies to mitigate and adapt to the impact of climate changes draws attention to how governments will reduce carbon emissions, promote energy conservation through alternative energy, encourage practices in food production and water preservation as part of the greater adaptation to disaster plans to improve resiliency and promote healthier lifestyles. Supporting resiliency remains a great challenge – with loss of income and crop failures related to droughts or flooding – in the region.

The widespread droughts in 2015 seen throughout the Americas were soon followed by the increase in vector-borne diseases in the region the following year. Further research continues since climate, vectors, and public health outcomes are influenced by such factors as temperature, rainfall, humidity, and altitude. Rising temperatures allow mosquitoes to survive in higher elevations and even crossing mountain ranges to appear as outbreaks in new regions, as seen in malaria in Kenya and Colombia. It is important to study climate and public health across the spatial and temporal shifts of pests and their pathogens as well as how human behaviors adapt with such changes taking place. Building resiliency will depend upon more vigorous policies and enforcements to protect human lives.

Disasters and Displacement

The good news is that we are seeing less deaths from disasters. The bad news is that there are greater economic losses today[34] which could have longer-term public health consequences. Weather-related events are causing the most displacement within LMICs. In 2016, 31.1 million people were displaced by disasters, violence, and conflict. A 2019 Internal Displacement Report revealed the highest number of displacements in history with 17.2 million newly displaced

Case Study 4.1

Cuba: Intersection of Disasters, Climate Change, Poor Infrastructure, and Infectious Diseases[17]

A disaster may not spontaneously trigger an outbreak of disease, unless, of course, a highly infectious disease is the reason for the emergency event. Nevertheless, a natural disaster will expose how vulnerable a country is to both newly emerging and reemerging communicable diseases when collapsing infrastructure, unable to support continuing neglect, threatens a nation. Cuba's challenges with cholera, dengue, and its viral relative, chikungunya, are good examples. Cholera and dengue spread throughout the island, while the Cuban government reported that all the cases of chikungunya were imported from Haiti and the Dominican Republic. Chikungunya, a viral disease transmitted by an infected mosquito, reached this hemisphere for the first time in history in December 2013 when it arrived on the Caribbean island of Saint Martin and spread throughout the region. Data revealed local transmission of chikungunya in 29 countries and territories in the Caribbean, Central, South, and North America, including the United States with a cumulative total of 508,122 suspected and 5,271 laboratory-confirmed cases, as of August 1, 2014.[18] Cuba rebuffs what independent journalists, rumors, and local health professionals describe on the island. The government's failure to release timely outbreak data will be discussed in later chapters on health diplomacy and health security. The relationship between climate change, failing infrastructure, and the frequency and intensity of natural disasters is considered in order to identify both the challenges and realities with re-emergence of infectious diseases of water-borne and vector-borne diseases such as cholera, dengue, and chikungunya. Cuba is a good case study since it has a well-developed epidemiologic surveillance system with highly skilled scientists and dedicated health professionals.

Climate Change

Scientists project climate change will continue to impact both the frequency and intensity of extreme weather patterns in the Caribbean. Islands like Cuba could expect rise in sea levels and this, combined with more intense weather events, will make flooding more common. Cuba's coastal regions will be impacted the most; however, Cuba could experience protracted seasons of both droughts and flooding, and reliable potable water could become scarce. According to José Rubiera, a leading Cuban Meteorologist, the "seawater temperature is rising and the conditions in the upper atmosphere are favourable to rapid intensification. These cases are now somewhat more frequent; it means something is changing."[19] The *vibrio cholera* bacteria has been known to survive in brackish waters and estuarine environments, attaches to zooplankton and moves along the ocean currents as it is carried into new areas,[20] continuing the threat to Cuba and Hispaniola. This danger is especially problematic in countries where fragile water, sanitation, sewage, and housing systems are further threatened by climate change and rising water temperatures where the multiplication of the cholera bacteria has been documented.[21]

Infrastructure

Earlier investment in the Cuban public health infrastructure is eroding quickly and without greater attention, the likelihood of increased risk of infectious diseases spreading spatially and temporally will continue. As reported in *The New England Journal of Medicine*, the reality is that, "Any visitor can see that Cuba remains far from a developed country in basic infrastructure such as roads, housing, plumbing, and sanitation."[22] According to ReliefWeb, the PAHO warned Cuba a week before Hurricane Sandy (October 2012) struck that further damage to the sanitation system could be problematic in the areas previously affected by cholera and other illnesses related to water use and handling of food. It is no surprise that "drinking water is contaminated in most Cuban cities," and neighborhoods have ongoing problems with sewage in the streets.[23] Let's not overlook the lack of hygienic supplies in hospitals and clinics. Cuban independent journalists along with dissident physicians have described water-borne and vector-borne disease outbreaks to be associated with the government's failure to meet basic sanitation standards.[24] Water treatment facilities seem to lack the chemicals, equipment, and appropriate filter units, along with the inconsistent availability of chlorine for safe water.[25] Furthermore, a failure to maintain continuous water pressure will hinder the amount of water and contribute to the contamination of the water supply.[26] Lastly, an engineering report on Cuba's infrastructure revealed "more than 50% of the water pumped through the distribution system is lost due to leaks in deteriorated piping."[27]

Natural Disasters

Based upon what we know about climate change and infrastructure demands in Cuba, the vulnerability and hazard reduction strategies associated with natural disasters are especially important with high winds, surging seas, and flooding. Hurricane season begins June 1 through November with October and November recognized as the most active times for hurricanes to strike in Cuba. The greatest risk for landslides is in the eastern provinces where earthquakes also have a higher likelihood of threats. While Cuba has a well-developed emergency evacuation and response plan, they show a poor performance in disaster reconstruction, recovery, and mitigation.[28] This is evident as a battered public health infrastructure continues to decline. According to researchers the most "troublesome is the lack of meaningful official programs to attempt to minimize or mitigate the damage that is caused by the severe vulnerability of the built environment to the hazard agents of hurricanes and earthquakes,"[29] Hurricanes Michelle (November 2001) and Isidore (September 2002) followed by Hurricane Lili (late September 2002) presented national challenges. However, it was Hurricanes such as Charley (August 2004) which became the most destructive to strike Cuba's western Havana region since 1914 followed by Hurricane Ivan (September 2004), the first Category 5 hurricane to hit Cuba in 80 years. This battered Pinar del Río, Cuba's westernmost province, which has been more regularly impacted by hurricanes. The 2005 hurricane season was very active with Hurricane Dennis (July), Hurricane Rita (September), and then Hurricane Wilma (October) reporting the worst death toll in Cuba in more than 40 years. After some quiet hurricane seasons, Hurricane Gustav (August 2008), a Category 4 hurricane, hit Cuba, and weeks after Tropical Storm Fay hit; Fay became the strongest storm in 60 years with an estimated $5 billion in damage to medical facilities, schools, infrastructure, crops, and livelihood.[30] Hurricane Ike (September 2008) reported hundreds of water wells in rural areas damaged, dams overflowing, and more than 1 million residents without potable water. U.S. engineers report that the "water supply system is unstable because pumps are in need of repair and because of frequent interruptions in the electrical supply needed to run the pumps,"[31] which is especially challenging during hurricane seasons. Hurricane Sandy (October 2012) hit the eastern region leaving devastation in Santiago de Cuba and Holguin while threatening highly populated communities and destroying critical public health infrastructure. In 2013, Ricardo Mena, a United Nations official responsible for disaster risk reduction in the Americas, announced that "Cuba has enormous amount of deteriorated buildings that can't withstand natural disasters."[32]

Conclusion

Rising sea levels, flooding, warming temperature, and the number and frequency of emergency events are expected to create more water-borne and vector-borne disease threats in contemporary times. Over the past decade, increasing risks and hazards on vulnerable populations present future challenges for Cuba and other Caribbean nations. Consequently, if Cuba's predicaments are related to climate change, re-occurring disasters, fragile infrastructure, economic or geopolitical reasons, or the intersection of all these factors, disasters could wreak havoc when nature calls[33] and Cuba is not alone.

people related to natural disasters and more specifically 1.7 million documented as weather-related events. The geography, typography, and lack of investments in mitigation strategies – with already weak infrastructure – place large numbers of people at risk. This is further complicated by the human factors of population growth, urbanization, land use, balance of resources, violence, and climate change with stresses on the environment disproportionately placing the most vulnerable populations.

One key strategy is to mitigate disasters using research on climate change. Nevertheless, even with the rigor of science, evidence-based decisions are not necessarily implemented. The reasoning spans from it is too costly to devote to something that may not happen again or so soon, to ideological differences and political expediency, which is especially relevant to the climate mitigation strategies for disasters. The value of research to improve community preparedness underscores how poverty, inequality, disease, and ill health thrive during emergency and post events. However, such findings need to be implemented before the next calamity strikes.

Disaster Response

In contemporary times, it is hard to keep up with the storms, hurricanes, flooding, and earthquakes wreaking havoc and not to forget the suffering of people behind the images of rubble and destruction. Once the cameras leave and the images fade, in what appears to be an attention-deficient disorder world, one emergency crisis will dominate the 24-hour news cycle until the next big event drives a fickle response. Many of the same communities are plummeted even before they have been able to get back to the pre-existing state prior to a previous event. This is exactly what happened in Ica, Peru where a 1998 mudslide devasted the region and seven years later a major earthquake struck the same communities.

Public health seeks to prevent and mitigate the suffering and avert a secondary disaster. A secondary disaster can be thought of in two ways. First, this refers to how an initial event, such as an earthquake, can cause buildings to collapse and trigger a secondary event from an electrical fire or release of toxic fumes. Second, it also refers to the human factors that produce or contribute to the crisis. A good example of this is the international response to Haiti's earthquake, which caused more than 200,000 deaths. This secondary event occurred when the Nepalese United Nations Peacekeeping Forces negligently dumped human waste into the Artibonite River, starting the catastrophic cholera epidemic that killed more than 9,000 people and up through 2018 more than 812,000 cases have been reported.[35] Cholera was able to spread rapidly due to the lack of public health infrastructure to protect the most vulnerable.

The secondary disasters I've observed are related to the best intentions to help in a post-disaster event. The dumping of supplies in countries, which are often not requested, and inappropriate, causes a drain on both personnel and resources to sort, discard, or find transport for delivery. Numerous hurricanes struck the Americas throughout the 1990s and 2000s and some of the university students volunteered to help sort through warehouse supplies prior to sending to the Caribbean and Central America. We found outdated medicines, improper clothing and undergarments, coats, and heavy sweaters during summer months, torn and worn shoes, and culturally unknown food products such as Jewish delicacies of matzah balls and gefilte fish somewhat like a fish meatloaf placed in glass jars along with weight reduction bars. In post-disaster events in different countries, I've seen how inappropriate supplies were either left in warehouses or in trash dumping sites. The call for donating money to reliable organizations remains the best practice. This could be local, national, or international not for profit organizations.[36]

On a Saturday at 11:30 am, January 13, 2001, an earthquake registering 7.6 on the Richter scale and subsequent landslides struck El Salvador, bringing about a secondary disaster, leaving more than 1 million homeless, 4,500 injured, 726 dead and an estimated 40–50% of the population without potable water. The coffee industry estimated its losses at $2.7 million, while the agricultural sector reported more than $130 million in damage. El Salvador declared that $1 billion would be needed to rebuild. Shortly after the event, I co-authored an opinion article for the "Miami Herald" with Carlos J. Castillo, then head of the International Miami-Dade County Search and Rescue Team, responding to Latin America and the Caribbean disasters, with an appeal to our community to not open their medicine cabinets or garages to send unrequested supplies to El Salvador; unless, of course, a well-coordinated path for receiving, storing, and distributing requested supplies was in place with local partnerships.

The most effective way to help victims from the devastating impact is to provide financial support to reliable agencies working with government organizations and NGOs. These agencies can establish clear mechanisms for the delivery and distribution of needed supplies and, equally important, can use the funds to buy goods, as available, in the affected country and stimulate the economy. Nevertheless, clothing, shoes, and food drives continue in post-disaster events.

As I finished writing this chapter, I return to add a message I just received from the Honduran American community collecting clothing, medicines, and food to send to Honduras in the aftermath of Hurricane Eta. Eta slammed through Central America on November 3, 2020, causing widespread flooding, destruction, and displacement from Panama to Guatemala, in the middle of the COVID-19 pandemic. Tragic reports and images of a wider humanitarian disaster are already motivating people to open their hearts and their closets. Once again, it is better to give money to trustworthy organizations working in the country, such as faith-based organizations with long experience working with local communities or *Cruz Roja* (Red Cross), among others, so they can best meet the needs of the population and their economy and not contribute to a secondary disaster.

Local-Level Capacity

Building local capacity is a best practice. The U.S. Agency for International Development, through the Office of U.S. Foreign Disaster Assistance, is responsible for coordinating all U.S. international disaster assistance. The goal is to build national and local self-sufficiency through investments in training, prevention, mitigation, and preparedness. During the mid-1980s through early 2000, the Miami-Dade Urban Search and Rescue team was one of two internationally trained U.S. teams (the other is in Fairfax, Virginia) that responded to more than 30 international disasters and trained almost 9,000 first responders. The success of that program was greatly credited to the in-country participation and bottom-up process used to develop training and technical assistance to local communities in Latin America and the Caribbean. The Miami-Dade team ensured that assistance was timely, culturally appropriate, necessary, and best utilized. Many of the first responders to the 2001 earthquake in El Salvador received technical assistance and training courses through Miami-Dade's department and where they learned that the most effective aid comes from within a country. While we see more intensity and frequency of disasters, the human impulse to help remains.

Local Capacity – Building Trust

A function of the University of Miami's Field Epidemiology Survey Team (FEST) was to conduct research and engage in disaster preparedness, response, and recovery work in collaboration with both first responders and communities. With a long history of working in remote communities with field appropriate tools, FEST adapted such skills to disaster projects. In 1985 Miami-Dade Fire Department (MDFD) initiated an agreement with the U.S. Federal Government, United States Agency for International Development Office of Foreign

Disaster Assistance to provide training for first responders on lifesaving rescue and advanced pre-hospital medical care following a disaster in Latin America and the Caribbean using locally available tools with the goal of self-sufficiency. In 1991, FEST Disaster Research Program began a collaboration with the Miami-Dade rescue team MDFD Florida Task Force 1 (FL-TF1) to help assess their efficiency and effectiveness during national and international disaster responses and training exercises. The purpose was to ensure that rescuers were doing the most they could without compromising their own health and safety. The agreement was conditioned that such evaluation would be used to improve the overall system of response, with input from different perspectives from administration, management, logistics, training, and field responders. This included assessments of their preparedness and response to hurricanes, tornadoes, earthquakes, plane crashes, terrorist events from 1991 to 2003.

FEST continued to adapt the field-based approaches to work with communities and NGOs in Latin America. For example, FEST's Disaster Research Program, in collaboration with World Vision, and local community partnerships, sought to assess community-based preparedness, mitigation, and response to emergency events in identified communities in Honduras, Nicaragua, and Ecuador. The community-based Central America Mitigation Initiative (CAMI, 2004) and the Community Emergency Response and Disaster Mitigation (CERDM 2006–2007) applied field-based assessments on administrative, training, logistical, and operational activities to identify the gaps and strengths from different stakeholders, and their perspectives. We were reminded that health, safety, and security start and end with the local community, as is the demand for public-private partnerships that respect and engage local public participation.

Case Study 4.2

Honduras Hurricane Mitch, 1998 – Public-Private Partnerships

In late October 1998, Hurricane Mitch struck Central America causing approximately 10,000 deaths. It made landfall on October 29, 1998 in Honduras, continuing to move slowly throughout Central America for the next few days with historic amounts of rainfall in Guatemala, Honduras, and Nicaragua causing great flooding. This became the second deadliest recorded hurricane in the Atlantic Ocean since the 1780 Great Hurricane of the West Indies where more than 20,000 deaths have been reported. With Hurricane Mitch, Honduras suffered the greatest impact leaving more than 5,000 dead, 2.8 million homes destroyed, and more than 2 million people evacuated. With 245 bridges destroyed and 133 damaged, it made search and rescue as well as a post–emergency response difficult. At the request of Honduran officials, a multidisciplinary team from Miami responded in the aftermath of Hurricane Mitch. We traveled to San Pedro Sula located in the northern part of Honduras close to the Caribbean coast. The city had an estimated population of 450,000, known as the industrial and commercial capital of Honduras. Our target area was located 17 km from San Pedro Sula in the city of La Lima, best known for the large banana plantations. The topography is flat, and the devastation caused by Hurricane Mitch was extensive.

This Honduras and United States collaborative response was multifaceted. It began with identifying the sites to distribute requested donated medical and health supplies; train local health workers on the use of field diagnostic kits in the rapid detection of malaria, dengue, and leptospirosis; and collaborate on technical support with local health professions and adapt public health educational tools for the post-disaster recovery. Most after-action meetings and subsequent reports highlighted improvements in national disaster plans, with an emphasis on finding ways to meet community needs. We proposed a plan to reinforce public-private partnerships and foster local capacity in disaster recovery.

Delivery of Technical Supplies and Medicine

One of the objectives of the Miami and Honduras collaborative response was to provide rapid diagnostic kits and the training of health professionals to use the kits in confirming suspected cases of malaria, dengue, and leptospirosis. A University of Miami microbiologist already working with Honduran counterparts in the northern region identified these as diseases of interest in a post-disaster event. Donations and low-cost purchase of rapid diagnostic kits were distributed between Social Security Hospital in San Pedro de Sula and La Lima Hospital. A training on the use of the rapid diagnostic kits in the field was conducted.[37]

Malaria

Malaria remains an important public health concern in Latin America and the Caribbean where it is endemic in 21 countries and territories and an estimated 100 million people are at risk. In 1997, researchers found increases in malaria and the more deadly form, Plasmodium falciparum, in northern Honduras. Such increases were due to longer rainy season, development of drug resistance, and cases being undiagnosed.[38] Rapid diagnostic tests were simple and easy to use. Rapid diagnostic kits for Malaria (OptiMal®) required three drops of blood obtained by a finger prick which was conducted by Honduran teams. Results of colored lines are visible within ten minutes.

This is important since in post-disaster settings many people assume that if they get a high fever it is malaria. And before a diagnostic confirmation is received people often resort to taking an anti-malarial drug. This has become a dangerous practice in the over utilization of chloroquine with risk to drug resistance. The purpose for this post-disaster response was not to conduct research but rather determine the advantages on the use of rapid diagnostic tools for point of care, which Honduran health providers found useful.

Dengue

Dengue continues to be an escalating public health issue in Latin America and the Caribbean and a leading cause of illnesses in some countries. A rapid diagnostic test for dengue was provided by PanBio® in Australia. The Honduran health team took blood samples mixed with a chemical to prevent the blood from clotting while it would sit for 30 minutes allowing blood plasma to separate from blood cells by natural gravity. One drop of plasma was placed on a nitrocellulose strip and allowed to migrate up the strip reacting with antibodies on the strip indicating a colored line if positive. This test took ten minutes and could tell if a person was infected (a primary infection) or had infection within the past few weeks with a previous dengue virus. The benefits of such dipsticks are that they are sensitive and specific in identifying a positive case of dengue, and provide information about people at risk for developing the potentially fatal Dengue Hemorrhagic Fever (DHF). The rapid test can be administered in the field without any equipment, and take only 40 minutes to run a test.

Leptospirosis

Malaria and dengue are well-known diseases in Latin America and the Caribbean, while the less known and greatly unreported leptospirosis is actually the most widespread zoonotic disease globally, as discussed in the globalization chapter. Climate change and flooding have contributed to its re-emergence throughout Central America. Human leptospirosis is acquired from direct or indirect exposure to urine of animals where rodents are the most important reservoir host. The signs of acute leptospirosis can range from influenza-like illness with chills, fever, headache, muscle ache, back pain, anorexia, nausea, and vomiting, which can be similar signs to many other diseases. Diagnosis is often difficult because the bacteria is not present very long in the blood and cultures take from two to three weeks to become positive. Donated Leptospira Dip-S-Ticks from Integrated Diagnostics, Inc. was a new diagnostic test at the time of Hurricane Mitch (1998). This test took two hours to run with plasma or serum. It is usually performed in a laboratory with samples incubating in a water bath for varying lengths of time. A dipstick with positive results appeared as a band across the dipstick. Honduran health providers and researchers found these tests to be beneficial in identifying cases.

Field Supportive Services

As with most major disasters, public health and safety needs are a priority. Families moved into *albergues* (disaster shelters), converted from schools, when they were displaced from their homes. Due to adverse living environments, newly displaced families had an increased risk of bacterial and viral infections as well as skin infections and infestation associated with lack of water and crowded conditions. At the United Farm Chiquita banana plantation, a hard-to-reach area obstructed by roads that were either washed away or flooded, travel and transport of supplies were difficult. Much of the population had lost their only source of income due to the destruction of banana crops. The MOH, using diagnostic tests, identified more cases of malaria and dengue in this area than in La Lima.

An infectious disease specialist was part of the Miami team collaborating with Honduran counterparts. Shelter visits found broken pipes in bathrooms and *aguas negras* (black standing water) due to rupture in the sewage pipes, raising many public health questions. High incidences of fever and diarrhea among children at the shelters were identified by the Health Department and La Lima Hospital and through the triage/ screening clinic at the shelter MOH, Hospital La Lima. Epidemiologic surveillance was conducted for dengue, malaria, and leptospirosis in collaboration with the MOH and Hospital La Lima. This supports why investments in community surveillance and the early provision of safe water, housing, and the protection of sewers remain the fundamental building blocks of public health safety in post-disaster situations.

Community Health Education

Along with the delivery of requested supplies, training on rapid diagnostics, and supportive health services, the collaboration included support through health education initiatives for disease prevention. We worked closely with the only health promoter in La Lima employed by the MOH, covering an estimated population of 130,000. The main focus was on potable drinking water and basic hygiene, which ranged from displayed posters, door-to-door visits, distribution of chlorine tablets, and education to mothers about the importance of clean drinking water.

In meeting with local partners, we discussed some previous public health work in post-disaster settings. One activity with wide interest was an educational tool that could be used for the start of the February 1999 school year, with financial and technical support through Northwest Medical Teams International, now Medical Teams International, and FEST to develop and implement the coloring and activity book with additional support through Volunteers in Technical Assistance (VITA), along with businesses and other nongovernmental agencies.

Post-Disaster Children's Pinta y Aprende Con Quique

In 1992 the devastation of Hurricane Andrew in Miami, Florida left many children afraid of another hurricane. A young educator working with Walt Disney volunteered her time and skills to collaborate with our team. I reached out to her once again to develop an activity book that could educate children and stimulate dialogue in a creative way for children aged 5–12. *Pinta y Aprende con Quique* (Draw and Learn with Quique) was a talking bird created with local heroes, local personnel, and a sense of familiarity for children. FEST had previous experience in developing culturally specific public health intervention tools in remote areas of Central and South America, including projects on community-based scabies elimination and control programs and a cholera prevention education program during the 1992 epidemic in Latin America, as well as simple data collection instruments for indigenous populations. The artist later developed coloring and activity books related to earthquakes, tornadoes, hurricanes, and terrorist events in collaboration with FEST (Figures 4.1 and 4.2)

Partnerships

A broad-based partnership was formed as shown in Table 4.1. This was built upon pre-existing relationships and additional funding awarded. To initiate the children's workbook project, focus groups from teachers,

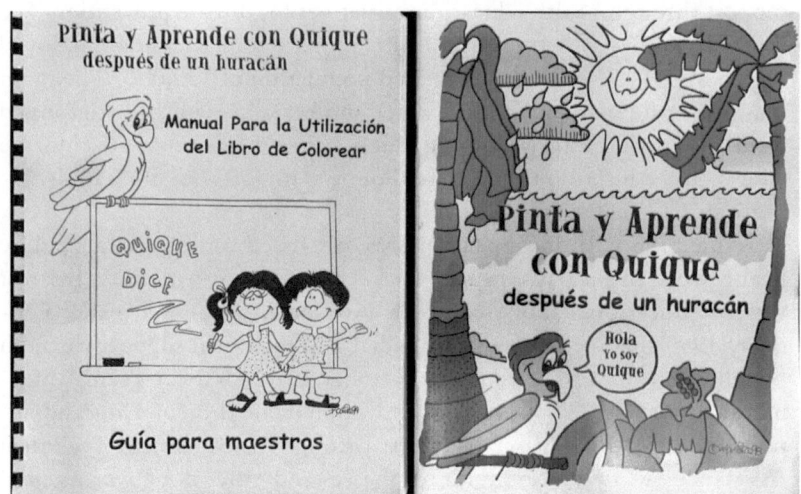

FIGURE 4.1 Post- Hurricane Mitch, Honduras: note: Teacher's Manual and Children's Workbook Teacher's Manual and Children's Workbook. *Pinta y Aprende Con Quique (Illustrations created by Karina Clark Rojas, 1999).*

children, community volunteers, librarians, nurses, and local doctors provide multiple perspective with list of topics on how to communicate appropriate health and safety messages with words and designs, and an educator's handbook to maximize the benefit. This included modules from simple messages for the younger children to geological and scientific and even physics activities for the older groups. The artist used the themes to provide preliminary sketches with input from the working group. Karina Rojas developed all drawings with the help of a graphic designer, and FEST collaborated with Honduran counterparts for the text content.

Evaluation and Local Ownership

Dr. Ada Rivera, Director of Preventive Medicine and Epidemiology at *Instituto Hondureño de Seguridad Social*, with extensive experience in community-based interventions and assessments for health and education tools in the region, led the project and the manual for teachers to optimize the use in schools. A feedback page was included with written or pictorial comments depending upon the age of the user. Modifications continued over a two-month period and from March 16 to 20, 1999 it was field tested and tweaked with final drawings, text, and

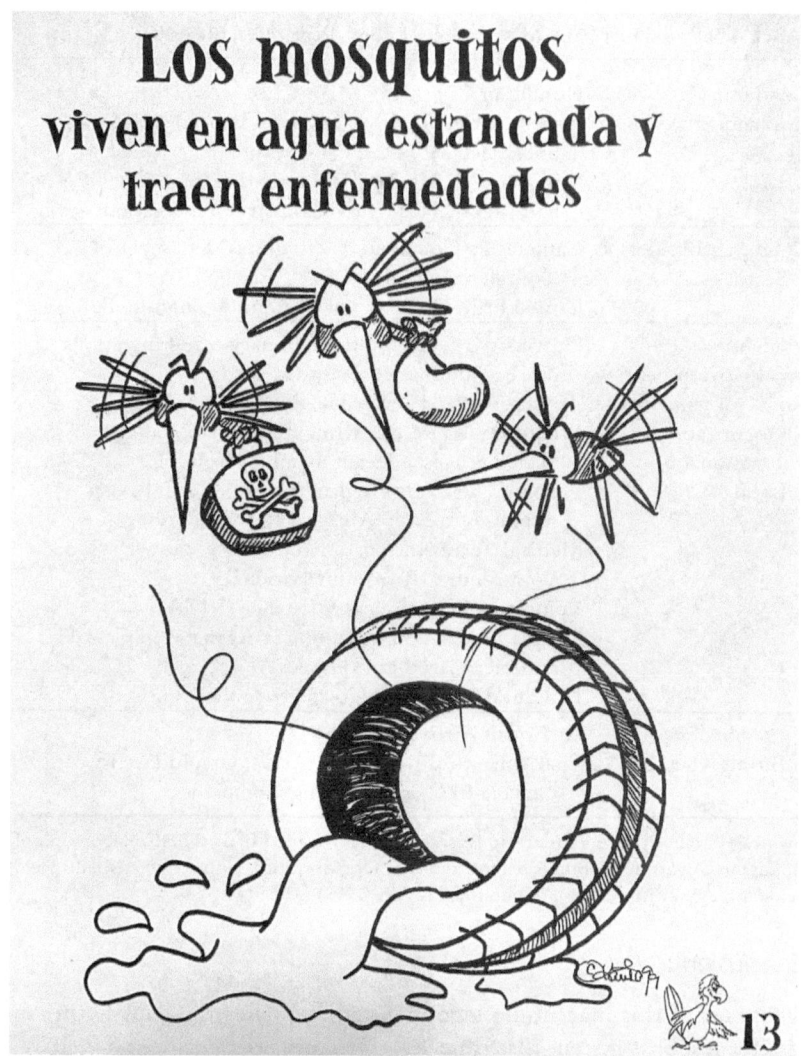

FIGURE 4.2 Post- Hurricane Mitch, Honduras: Public Health Message Mosquitoes live in standing water and carry diseases. *Pinta y Aprende Con Quique (Illustrations created by Karina Clark Rojas, 1999).*

feedback. The teacher's manual, consisting of three educational modules from kindergarten to grade six, also came to fruition through the public-private partnership. This became a locally owned project with wider reach.

TABLE 4.1 Post-Hurricane Mitch – The Public-Private Partnerships

Honduran Government	Honduran Consulate (Miami)
	Instituto Hondureño de Seguridad Social (IHSS) – Social Security Hospital Institute
	Ministerio de Salud y Ministerio de Educación - Ministry of Health and Ministry of Education
Honduran Business Sector	Camaras de Comercio de Honduras- Chamber of Commerce Honduras
	United Fruit Company of Honduras (Chiquita Banana)
Academia Local Government Non-Governmental Organizations International to Local	University Miami multidisciplinary team: infectious disease, international studies, medicine, microbiology, and public health
	Miami Dade Fire Department/International Urban Search & Rescue team members from Florida Task Force 1 with experience in logistics and disaster responses to Latin America and the Caribbean.
	Medical Teams International formerly known as North West Medical Team International
	Volunteers in Technical Assistance (VITA)/ Florida Association of Volunteer Agencies in Central America Caribbean (FAVACA)
	Honduras Manos Amigo and Save the Children.
United States Business Sector	American Airlines,
	Pharmaceutical Donations, Artist, Graphic Artist, Crayola LLC, and Printing Companies.

Source: A Public-Private Partnership Response to Hurricane Mitch: The Collaboration of Honduran Government, Public Sector, and U.S. Organizations. University of Miami Field Epidemiology Team (FEST), unpublished report (1999)

Conclusion

A disaster of this magnitude identifies and augments the gaps within a disaster response system that is necessary to meet the health and welfare of the most vulnerable populations. The devastation of this hurricane required more than local government involvement; while people needed to become part of the process in rebuilding their lives, as well as understanding mitigation strategies to become more resilient for future events. This is where global public–private partnerships can be valuable.

A Disaster System of Response

While governments are ultimately responsible for the health and welfare of its people, we've seen unequal governmental responses throughout the region. What we do observe is the growth of NGOs, faith-based, citizen groups, and public-private partnerships to provide aid in a post-disaster event. There are numerous stories to be told about untrained or disaster tourists showing up in a Latin America or Caribbean country because they saw the devastation on the television, blog, or other social media platforms. They arrive unprepared and can often become a drain on limited local resources. There are many well-meaning people and organizations that want to offer assistance, and I cannot think of a better example than what took place in the Caribbean during the response to the 2010 earthquake in Haiti. I suggest that the story I share below is not intended to be unique to Haiti and it could have happened elsewhere.

Case Study 4.3

Public-Private Partnerships: Haiti Earthquake, January 2010

Haiti, once a rich French colony, has become the poorest country in the Western Hemisphere. It is situated in the Caribbean on the island of Hispaniola, which it shares with Dominican Republic to the east, surrounded by Puerto Rico and the countries of Cuba and Jamaica. Even though it shares the same island, Haiti is a French and Creole speaking country while Dominicans speak Spanish. The social, cultural, economic, environmental, and political situations are also quite different. Haiti's statistics feature the inextricable relationship of the social determinants of health resulting in devastating outcomes for the country. However, it is the tragedies associated with colonialism, neoliberalism, globalization, climate change, droughts and increasing hurricanes, vast environmental degradation that provide a more in-depth view of Haiti's situation today.

Haiti has become one of the world's most unequal countries, with a widening gap of income distribution, and the growing urban and rural disparities. The lack of public health infrastructure is evident with 52% of the rural population living without access to safe drinking water, all while infectious diseases continue at a high rate such as diarrhea and typhoid, malaria, and dengue fever. The bleak social, economic, and political situations are further complicated by their geography and environmental factors.

Earthquake and Secondary Disaster

Haiti is also situated in a region prone to earthquakes and hurricanes. Yet, Haiti was wholly unprepared for the 2010 devastating earthquake.

The outdated building codes and lack of enforcement, in part, explain how 300,000 homes and 180 government buildings collapsed or were severely damaged; 1.5 million people became homeless; 50% of the hospitals were destroyed or seriously damaged, along with 80% of the schools and the destruction of the major port, roads, and economic system.[39] The disaster risk to an already vulnerable population is exacerbated by the persistent hazards of Haiti's deforestation and soil erosion. The 2008 hurricane season left Haiti evermore fragile. And the catastrophic earthquake that struck on January 12, 2010 at 4:53 pm with its epicenter just 25 km from the capital city of Port-au-Prince was more than the country could handle. As a result, international humanitarian aid rushed in. This was followed by the secondary disaster, a deadly cholera outbreak, which continued to wreak havoc on the health of an already suffering nation. According to the Centers for Disease Control and Prevention (2018), there were approximately 820,000 cases of cholera in Haiti with more than 9,000 deaths reported.

There is a lot of blame to go around, but this case study is not about blame, nor specifically about the earthquake or the cholera outbreak. It will not cover the political issues, corruption, or the role of Nepalese United Nations Peacekeeping Forces bringing cholera to Haiti during the post-earthquake period. Rather, it opens the door to the wider discussion of missteps in international humanitarian aid, presented through a specific occurrence during the post-earthquake Haiti response.

Public-Private Partnerships in Disasters

The purpose of this case study is to draw the reader's attention to a gap in the international emergency response system, especially in the delivery and intent of foreign aid to the resource poor nation of Haiti. The call for public-private partnerships, with the best of intentions and sincere desire to reduce human suffering, exposes a variety of unintended consequences. Haiti is reported to have more international NGOs per square footage than any other country in the world and is sometimes referred to as the Republic of NGOs. The varying estimates suggest up to 10,000 NGOs are working in the country. There is a much bigger story about how good or bad this is for Haiti, but that discussion I leave for Haitian people to explore.

The worst natural disaster wreaked havoc on an already poverty stricken Haiti exposing stark inequalities. The devastation was shared around the globe with graphic images of the desperate cries for loved ones and neighbors buried under the mountains of rubble and debris.

Traditional and social media expanded the reach to new audiences, covering different perspectives about the arrival of donations and foreign aid supplies rolling into the country to help victims and their families survive and rebuild. While the earthquake and secondary disaster of the cholera epidemic have been discussed extensively in the literature, I'd like to tell the story of one businessman who responded in what he claims was a humanitarian call to save Haitian lives and limbs. I present this story, with the permission and eagerness of this businessman to impart his experience about volunteerism and the business sector's contribution during a post-disaster event; however, I've chosen to use the pseudonym, Steve, for purposes of this case study.[40]

Private Sector in Disaster Response

Steve matches uninsured or underinsured people with health and travel insurance and likes to say he is in the business of helping people. A few days after the Haiti earthquake struck one of his clients, who manufactures a wireless battery-operated digital X-ray machine, offered to donate the 900-pound $250,000 machine to Haiti. Steve knew he had to find a way to get it there as quickly as possible. Living in Texas, he along with the X-ray company's service engineer, flew with the machine and equipment to Miami. They transported it into a flatbed truck to the Homestead Airforce Base, south of Miami, to wait for an aircraft to take them to the capital city of Port-au-Prince. They boarded a military C-131 aircraft 24 hours later and shortly thereafter, they landed upon a dark runway in the middle of the night. The machine was offloaded and together they traveled to the Port-au-Prince hospital where it was operational by 8:00 am. According to Steve, this was the only X-ray machine available at that time, so all the health providers were eager to use it to pinpoint the fractured bones, especially those of the children.

Steve remained in Haiti for 22 days, 17 days of which he participated in taking X-rays, while holding the hands of the traumatized injured children. He recounted how during the first few days they took thousands of digital X-rays, and from January to April 2010 approximately 33,000 X-rays were taken. At a glance this story profiles both humanitarianism and the indomitable human spirit to seek fast solutions to reach the unmet needs. However, it also exposes the important lessons about public health and safety protocols and the oversight that is necessary for a disaster response system to work for all. I first met Steve in 2010 and he shared his amazing feat to arrive with this digital X-ray machine so soon after the earthquake struck. The more we talked, the more he felt comfortable sharing another side of the story. When they offloaded the first box of the digital machine and connective supplies, the second box, which contained the lead screens and lead vests, did not follow along.

The service engineer reminded Steve that he had to maintain distance to prevent even a very low-dose exposure to radiation. He said he understood. Nevertheless, when the young, frightened children arrived, many without a parent or a surviving family member, he disregarded the protection of his own health and safety. As he told me, "I chose to hold the hands of the kids to offer comfort." He continued this for days that turned into more than two weeks. Ultimately, Steve started to feel sick with headaches, nausea, and fatigue symptoms, and he assumed that he, "picked up some bug" during his stay. Feeling worse, he made plans to return home and seek out medical attention. He hitched a ride on a C-17 Air Force plane and landed in Orlando, Florida where a bus took him to the Orlando Airport. Feeling worse, he decided to stay at a hotel for three days before heading back home to Texas. Feeling somewhat better, he still thought it would be best to see his health care provider.

Volunteerism and Health Consequences

Based upon Steve's account, his concerned physician identified a very low red blood cell count and referred him to an oncologist. Due to his recent history and exposures, the specialist referred him to a radiologist who, in turn, diagnosed his condition as radiation poisoning from the repeated exposure. He was treated by a hematologist and started to feel better.

However, in January 2012 Steve began to have eye problems, and by March 2012 he experienced vision loss in his right eye and diminishing vision in his left. After many doctor consultations and diagnoses, he ended up traveling to Ireland for a very successful cornea surgery related to his radiation exposure.

Thinking this was behind him, with no other related symptoms, things changed exactly two years later to the month. In March 2014, Steve felt as if his teeth were falling out of his mouth. He immediately visited his dentist, who then referred him to an oral surgeon. The diagnosis was severe jawbone deterioration. What was the cause? He recounted how an oral surgeon diagnosed radiation absorption of the jawbone, a condition called osteoradionecrosis. By now Steve became well voiced in the medical jargon and continued to recite scientific terms that crossed his many different health conditions, all of which I had to look up in writing this case study. This was four years after his extended low-dose exposures in the aftermath of the Haiti earthquake. His treatment was hyperbaric oxygen for five days a week, four times a day, over a period of eight weeks. Fortunately, he was able to continue the same protocol in his home state of Texas. While this helped, he continued to suffer chronic pain. He shared that this all changed at a dinner party when he fortuitously met a world-renowned pioneering scientist and physician from Munich, Germany, known for his stem cell work. In the words of Steve, "he saved my life."

Discussion

This story reveals the benefits and drawbacks of a disaster response system that is not well defined or implemented. On the harmful side it exposed the lack of oversight and training for the health and safety protocols for non-health workers responding to an international disaster. The requirements of training have not been fully realized. Second, it demonstrates a lack of inclusion of the public and private sectors in a well-defined international emergency response system where supply chain management plays a key role. If he only had the lead screen, would his life be much different? Lastly, it exposes the unintended negative health consequences of humanitarian efforts among untrained participants. The positive side is that this X-ray machine provided the diagnostic tool needed for the rapid detection of the many painful broken bones requiring surgery. It also showed the willingness of global citizens to mobilize both resources and actions to deliver a highly prized machine to the front lines. This is where global public-private partnerships for disasters have gained great momentum.

I've seen many needed supplies land in places left with no one at the other end to collect or transport due to lack of available transportation, poor roads, and collapsed bridges. Here the logistical management of a supply chain within a fragmented system of disaster response once again exposes a major gap in the system when the digital X-ray machine with imaging and computer adapters arrived, while the protective screens were left somewhere behind. That is why a logistician and a loadmaster, who is responsible for safely loading, transporting, and unloading supplies on a military or civilian aircraft, are essential roles within a well-defined and coordinated disaster response system. This is an important lesson for all responders, from professionals to volunteers that the individual organizations and groups are only as good as the system can support. We often blame governments, individuals, organizations, etc.; yet we fail to scrutinize the system of response where equal gaps across the training, education, management, administration, logistics, and response must be seamless and accountable.

Conclusion

What is clear, Steve encountered great misfortune. It is not clear and obvious if his post-health issues were all directly related to the radiation exposure. I take him at his word with his meticulous details about his health and medical situation. It would not matter to Steve, anyway. He was eager to tell me, "I'd do it all over again if I was in the same situation." His words are important to hear since Steve continues to lend his service during other emergency events. This is especially crucial, as we have seen throughout this chapter that an increase in the intensity and frequency of disasters in Latin America and the Caribbean threatens the region. I would like to think, if he did do it over again, he would be better prepared to prevent this from happening again, and if not, that the system would be better prepared to provide the oversight necessary to protect such compassionate volunteers. It will take a more robust coordinated system of response of training and engaging public-private partnerships to prevent a similar situation happening again.

Disasters: Public-Private Partnerships – Peru Earthquake 2007

On August 15, 2007, at 6:40 pm local time, a 7.9 earthquake struck off the coast of Peru, south of Lima. Over 500 people died in the quake and nearly 20,000 homes were completely destroyed. The cities of Pisco, Chincha, and Ica were impacted as the small towns and communities suffered greatly. Tragically, these same communities had been struggling since 1998 from a series of disastrous mudslides. Richard Weisskoff, Professor and Chairperson of the Department of International Studies, at the University of Miami was working with the Ica community on dam and tree planting to mitigate further mudslide devastation. Five weeks before the earthquake I traveled with Weisskoff, as part of a two-year project to address the unmet needs dated back to the 1998 mudslides. It was El Niño that brough heavy rainfall and flooding to Peru in 1997–1998, causing major land erosion, which triggered the mudslides and rise in food insecurity, and nutritional impact on newborns during that time. The projects were initiated just prior to the 2007 earthquake. On the day it struck, local representatives for the collaborative Peru projects were hosting a community forum to provide children with school uniforms and establish small businesses for economic community initiatives. The earthquake left them stranded forcing them to walk hours to return to their homes.

Two weeks after the earthquake, with an invitation from local officials, we participated in damage assessment within the Los Molinos, Ica region, in collaboration with local partners. A systematic collection of feedback from people in the affected area was designed to identify immediate and long-term needs among the target population, discuss the small-scale economic development projects, and expand the network with the local government and community leaders for long-term sustainability.

Through a collaboration with the local community government, teachers, engineers, and nongovernment partners, we devised a simple and easy to use multifaceted survey that collected information on housing, education levels, water source and usage, sanitation, garbage, pests, health and health access, employment, and animal and land inventory. This survey instrument was field tested the first day in the small community and modified based upon the input from community members. Implemented two weeks post disaster 52 families with 199 individuals, 53% male and 47% female, were surveyed. Some selected public health findings showed that 87% of the homes suffered moderate or major damage and 51% were destroyed with 43% living in a tent and 23% living in a shack, while 25% chose to remain in their severely damaged home. Residents stated their water was cloudy, dirty, bad tasting, and almost 50% indicated odor. Yet 75% said they were not treating drinking water and 25% used tablets to treat their water, which was given to them from the foreign aid teams. This included Germany, Ireland, Red Cross, and a Japanese medical team. The government and local partners used the information to improve upon short-term interventions.[41]

Over decades of field work, I have also learned to appreciate the value of listening to people to systematically collect key words they use to describe how they see their situation. Today we use computer-generated word cloud graphics to depict the terms or expressions that resonate with an audience. Back then, no such programs existed; nevertheless, the importance then and now remains. When people were asked to describe in their own words how they felt after the earthquake, the prevailing themes were sad, scared, frightened, nervous, and poor. These words were incorporated into the community dialogues as ideas emerged for economic development activities and inter-community collaboration with mitigation and resiliency plans as part of the larger rebuilding effort, ensuring the voices of the victims were heard. Local engineer, Roberto Navarro, promoted small sustainable development projects beyond the investment of foreign aid for disaster recovery and focused on microbusiness loans and activities to meet local needs. Things happen best when the local community maintains the ownership of their projects with measurable objectives.

Concluding Remarks

Mitigating disasters and building resiliency from earthquakes, extreme weather, climate change droughts and flooding, fires, landslides, and hurricanes require greater inquiry into the interaction of more than people and the environment. Further study of planetary health and disasters could create a wider space to examine how human systems will respond to such stresses as the unstable balance of people, animals, plants, and microbes in the ecosystem continues as germane to the discussion. It was Paul Crutzen, the 1995 Dutch Nobel Prize recipient in chemistry who first coined the term Anthropocene in 2000. He presented this new geological epoch to exemplify how human activities were impacting the global effect on earth's systems. Biophysical changes are disrupting global climate systems leading to the pollution of water, air, and soil, with biodiversity losses, changes in land use and land cover, and resource scarcity of freshwater and arable land,[42] which will continue to impact many populations.

We recognize health outcomes have improved, while our ecosystem has not. How humanity is expected to keep pace with declining ecological and biophysical changes suggests greater investments in ecosystem sustainability. This includes embracing the value of sustainable science, "the interaction between natural and social systems, and with how these interactions affect the challenge of sustainability; meeting the needs of present and future generations while substantially reducing poverty and conserving the planet's life support systems."[43] Sustainable science provides a compelling argument for further inquiry into the interconnectedness of disasters, climate crisis, displacement, planetary health, and the safety and security of populations moving forward. It also offers an opportunity to further connect different academic disciplines and establish best practices in the prevention, mitigation, preparedness, response, and rebuilding for a more resilient society that will respect and protect people and the planet. We need to do better.

Notes

1 Pan American Health Organization and World Health Organization, *Climate Change and Health in Small Island Developing States: A WHO Special Initiative in Collaboration with UNFCCC and the Fijian Presidency of the COP-23 – SIDS in the Caribbean Region* (Washington, DC: PAHO, 2018), https://www.paho.org/hq/index.php?option=com_docman&view=download&category_slug=technical-reports-9862&alias=46262-climate-change-and-health-in-small-island-developing-states-1&Itemid=270&lang=en.
2 Kevin E. Trenberth et al., "Global Warming and Changes in Drought," *Nature Climate Change* 4 (2014): 17–22, doi:10.1038/nclimate2067.
3 John C. Burnham, "A Neglected Field: The History of Natural Disasters," *Perspectives on History* (1988), https://www.historians.org/publications-and-directories/perspectives-on-history/april-1988/a-neglected-field-the-history-of-natural-disasters.
4 Office of US Foreign Disaster Assistance, *Disaster History: Significant Data on Major Disasters Worldwide, 1900-Present* (Washington, DC: Agency for International Development, 1993).
5 William Chester Jordan, *The Great Famine: Northern Europe in the Late Fourteenth Century* (Princeton, NJ: Princeton University Press, 1996).

6 Pitirim A. Sorokin, *Man and Society in Calamity* (New York: E. P. Dutton & Co., 1942).
7 Stuart B. Schwartz, *Sea of Storms a History of Hurricanes in the Greater Caribbean from Columbus to Katrina* (Princeton, NJ: Princeton University Press, 2015).
8 "The Global Historical Context of Emergency Management," Session 3 of FEMA's Comparative Emergency Management Course. The Training Material Can Be Accessed Here: https://training.fema.gov/hiedu/docs/cem/comparativeemcourse-session3-theglobalhistoricalcontextofemergencymanagement.doc.
9 Greg Bankoff, "Historical Concepts of Disaster and Risk," in *Handbook of Hazards and Disaster Reduction*, eds. Ben Wisner, JC Gaillard, and Ilan Kelman (New York: Routledge, 2011), 37–47.
10 "Vulnerability," United Nations Development Program, 2004.
11 World Economic Forum, *The Global Risks Report* (Cologny: World Economic Forum, 2019).
12 Gerardo Suárez and Virginia García-Acosta, *The Seismic Alert System in Mexico City: An Example of a Successful Early Warning System (EWS)*, Case Studies Series (Geneva: UNISDR Scientific and Technical Advisory Group, 2014).
13 Jonathan Stone et al., *Integrating Community and Observatory Based Monitoring to Reduce Risk at Volcán Tungurahua, Ecuador*, Case Studies Series (Geneva: UNISDR Science and Technical Advisory Group, 2014).
14 UNISDR Scientific and Technical Advisory Group, *Case Study 10: Building Resilience to Earthquakes in Chile* (Report) (Geneva: UNISDR, 2013), https://www.preventionweb.net/files/workspace/7935_casestudy10.pdf.
15 Jacqueline Charles, "Bahamas Has No Idea of Dorian Death Toll after Names of the Missing Were Removed from List," *The Miami Herald*, June 12, 2020.
16 Jason Von Meding, David O Prevatt, and Ksenia Chmutina, "Dorian's Destruction in the Bahamas Rooted in Historic Inequality in the Bahamas" (op-ed), *The Miami Herald*, December 16, 2019.
17 Portions of this case study have been published online through the University of Miami's Institute of Cuban and Cuban American Studies (ICCAS): Focus on Cuba. See Sherri L. Porcelain, "When Nature Calls: Cuba's Public Health Infrastructure Exposed," *ICCAS: Focus on Cuba*, Web/Issue 222, August 14, 2015.
18 Centers for Disease Control and Prevention, *Chikungunya in the Americas*, accessed August 8, 2014, http://www.cdc.gov/chikungunya/geo/americas.
19 Patricia Grogg, "Q&A: Hurricanes are Getting Stronger in the Caribbean" (Interview with José Rubiera), *InterPress Service*, July 10, 2013, http://www.ipsnews.net/2013/07/qa-hurricanes-are-getting-stronger-in-the-caribbean/.
20 Rita R. Colwell, "Global Climate Change and Infectious Disease: The Cholera Paradigm," *Science* 274, no. 5295 (1996): 2025–2031, doi:10.1126/science.274.5295.2025.
21 Joan L. Aron and Johnathan Patz, *Ecosystem Change and Public Health: A Global Perspective* (Baltimore, MD: Johns Hopkins University Press, 2001).
22 Edward D. Campion and Stephen Morrissey, "Perspective: A Different Model-Medical Care in Cuba," *New England Journal of Medicine* 368 (2013): 297–299.
23 Katherine Hirschfeld, "Book Review: Linda Whiteford and Laurence Branch, *Primary Health Care in Cuba*: The Other Revolution, Lanham: Rowman and Littlefield, 2008," *Society* 46 (2009): 294.
24 Ibid.
25 Manuel Cereijo and Helena M. Solo-Gabriele eds., *Infrastructure Assessment for a Transition in Cuba (March 11, 2011)* (Miami: The Endowment for Cuban American Studies, 2008), 11.
26 Ibid.
27 Ibid, 12.

28 B. E. Aguirre and Joseph E. Trainor, "Emergency Management in Cuba: Disasters Experienced, Lessons Learned, and Recommendations for the Future," in *Comparative Emergency Management: Understanding Disaster Policies, Organizations, and Initiatives from Around the World*, ed. David A. McEntire (Washington, DC: FEMA, 2009), https:// training.fema.gov/hiedu/aemrc/booksdownload/compemmgmtbookproject.

29 Ibid, 5.

30 Canadian Red Cross, *Cuba Hurricanes 2008*, accessed August 7, 2014, https:// www.redcross.ca/how-we-help/current-emergency-responses/past-emergency-responses/past-emergencies-and-disasters/international/2008/hurricanes-2008/ cuba-hurricanes-2008.

31 Helena M. Solo-Gabriele and Armando I. Perez, "Cuba's Water and Wastewater Sector: Environmental Literature, Institutional and Economic Issues and Future Work," *Association for the Study of the Cuban Economy* 18 (November 30, 2008): 383, 378–389 https://www.ascecuba.org/asce_proceedings/cubas-water-and-wastewater-sector-environmental-literature-institutional-and-economic-issues-and-future-work/

32 Jean Friedman-Rudovsky, "Hurricane Tips From Cuba," *The New York Times*, July 30 2013, D.6.

33 Sherri L. Porcelain, "When Nature Calls."

34 Centre for Research on the Epidemiology of Disasters, *Natural Disasters 2017* (Brussels: CRED, 2018), https://reliefweb.int/report/world/natural-disasters-2017.

35 Pan American Health Organization and the World Health Organization, *Epidemiological Update: Cholera* (Washington, DC: PAHO/WHO, 2018).

36 Note: Charity Navigator was founded in 2001 and today they evaluate hundreds of thousands of charitable organizations that have offices in the U.S. See https:// www.charitynavigator.org/. CharityWatch was founded in 1992 and it evaluates religious charities and social welfare groups from grades A to F. See https://www. charitywatch.org/. GuideStar, run by Candid, was created in 1994 and provides information for donors to make informed decisions on where to donate. See https:// www.guidestar.org/. While there are many others, these are useful tools for the decision-making process about where to donate money.

37 The information presented below is based upon a 1999 unpublished joint report from the University of Miami and Honduran partnerships in response to Hurricane Mitch.

38 Carol J. Palmer, et al., "Increased Prevalence of *Plasmodium Falciparum* Malaria in Honduras, Central America," *Revista Panamericana de Salud Pública* 4, no. 1 (1998): 40–42, http://www.scielosp.org/scielo.php?script=sci_arttext&pid=S1020-49891998000700007&lng=pt&nrm=iso&tlng=en.

39 Reginal DesRoches et al., "Overview of the 2010 Haiti Earthquake," *Earthquake Spectra* 27, no. S1 (2011): S1–S21, https://escweb.wr.usgs.gov/share/mooney/142. pdf.

40 Skype Interviews with author, March 2011, and Zoom follow-up interview, May 20, 2020.

41 The information presented is based upon a 2007 unpublished report compiled for Los Molinos, Ica Regional Office, Peru in the post-earthquake response.

42 Samuel S. Meyers, "Planetary Health: Protecting Human Health in a Rapidly Changing Planet, *The Lancet* 390, no. 10114 (2017): 2869–2868, doi:10.1016/ S0140-6736(17)32846-5.

43 Robert W. Kates, "What Kind of a Science Is Sustainability Science?," *Proceedings of the National Academy of Science* 108, no. 49 (2011): 19449–19450, doi:10.1073/ pnas.1116097108. Quoted in Didier Wernli et al., "Moving Global Health Forward in Academic Institutions," *Journal of Global Health* 6, no. 1 (2016): 3.

Bibliography – Selected Books

Button, Gregory. *Disaster Culture: Knowledge and Uncertainty in the Wake of Human and Environmental Catastrophe*. Walnut Creek, CA: Taylor and Francis, 2016.

Crosby, Alfred W. *Ecological Imperialism: The Biological Expansion of Europe, 900–1900*. Cambridge: Cambridge University Press, 2004.

Emmanuel, Kerry. *Divine Wind. The History and Science of Hurricanes*. Oxford: Oxford University Press, 2005.

Erlick, June Carolyn. *Natural Disasters in Latin America and the Caribbean: Coping with Calamity*. New York: Routledge, 2021.

Jordan, William Chester. *The Great Famine: Northern Europe in the Late Fourteenth Century*. Princeton, NJ: Princeton University Press, 1996.

Lemery, Jay and Auerback, Paul. *Enviromedics: The Impact of Climate Change on Human Health*. Washington, DC: Rowan & Littlefield, 2017.

Levy, Barry and Patz, Jonathan. *Climate Change and Public Health*. New York: Oxford University Press, Incorporated, 2015.

McMichael, Anthony J. *Planetary Overload: Global Environmental Change and the Health of the Human Species*. Cambridge: Cambridge University of Press, 1993.

Myers, Samuel and Frumkin, Howard. *Planetary Health: Protecting Nature to Protect Ourselves*. Washington, DC: Island Press, 2020.

Noji, Eric K., ed. *The Public Health Consequences of Disasters*. Oxford: Oxford University Press, 1997.

O'Mathúna, Dónal P, Dranseika, Vilius, and Gordijn, Bert. *Disasters: Core Concepts and Ethical Theories. Advancing Global Bioethics*. Cham: Springer, 2018.

Rigby, Catherine E. *Dancing with Disaster: Environmental Histories, Narratives, and Ethics for Perilous Times*. Acls Humanities E-Book. Charlottesville: University of Virginia Press, 2015.

Schwartz, Stuart B. *Sea of Storms: A_History of Hurricanes in the Greater Caribbean from Columbus to Katrina*. Princeton, NJ: Princeton University Press, 2015.

5

HEALTH DIPLOMACY

Negotiating community health activities and policies has been controversial throughout history. Polarized judgments underscore the different actors' points of view, whether their priority is based on protecting people, animals, ecosystem, economy, or geopolitical reasons. The ascent to contemporary health diplomacy shows the range of perspectives from humanitarianism, social justice, human rights, development, to a more security centric approach. This has legitimized the global health shift from low to high politics and where diplomacy offers a broader political agenda for transnational border cooperation.

As noted throughout this book, language matters. This is equally true in uniting terms of diplomacy and public health. Diplomacy is defined as the art, science, and practice of conducting international relations as an instrument used by actors to promote and implement their foreign policy interests.[1] It recognizes that "[T]he art of diplomacy juggles with the science of public health and concrete national interest balances with the abstract collective concern of the larger international community in the face of intense lobbying and advocacy."[2] According to Adams, Novotny, and Leslie, the term global health diplomacy identifies political shifts to meet shared health goals by strengthening relationships to fulfill the resource gaps.[3] Katz et al. show how health diplomacy has progressed from the traditional forms of nation-state interactions that produce bilateral and multilateral agreements and treaties to include more participation of multistakeholders and nonstate actors, as well as the extension of informal levels of diplomacy that take place today.[4] Kickbush et al. demonstrate how the practice of diplomacy is not necessarily about diplomat-to-diplomat relations and today negotiations will include more involvement from nongovernmental organizations, scientists,

DOI: 10.4324/9781003007401-6

activists, and private entities. Health diplomacy seeks to capture multi-level and multi-actor negation processes to shape and manage the global policy environment for health.[5]

What is noteworthy is that health diplomacy can take place at local, national, regional, and global levels. Nevertheless, the challenge and relevancy of diplomatic actions to influence population health, safety, and security will need local and national commitments. As diplomacy is fundamental to public health, it is unfortunately misinterpreted. The term health diplomacy has become conflated with the portrayal of medical diplomacy; therefore, it deserves further clarity. Medical diplomacy has its origins in the mobilization of doctors and other allied professionals to countries to fill existing gaps in their medical care services; or more often during disasters or other emergency events that weaken a country's ability to meet their population needs. Since the 1959 Cuban Revolution, Cuba has become the most recognized country in the world for its medical diplomacy, generating 60 years of good will for their South to South exchange of doctors for oil or mobilizing doctors to country for cash. Cuba's investment in creating large numbers of doctors, nurses, and allied health professionals was the expression of Fidel Castro's revolution. Using health professionals as a form of diplomacy was embraced early in the formation of the new Cuban government, sending medical missions to Algeria during their civil war with France, while Cuba provided aid early in 1960. In 1963 Cuba's medical and health technical assistance to Africa began with 29 doctors, 3 dentists, 15 nurses, and 8 medical technicians.[6] From 1961 to 2008 Cuba reported working in more than 154 countries with health workers in 70 countries.[7] Mobilizing such medical aid to resource poor countries was central to Castro's post-revolution foreign policy,[8] and portrays the image of medical diplomacy.

Peter Bourne, special assistant for health issues under President Jimmy Carter, introduced the concept of medical diplomacy in 1978 into the wider discussion of international relations. However, the term transitioned into health diplomacy with changes in the interactions of research, policy, and increased public-private partnerships for global health. This chapter will focus on the aspects of health diplomacy as a necessary step to achieve health security in Chapter 6. I present examples and case studies to explore the trajectory of health diplomacy through transborder strategies in the Americas.

Historical Context

International relations scholars identify the 1648 Treaty of Westphalia as the origin of international governance that gave states their sovereignty to establish policies within their border. This included pioneering new laws intrinsic to the health and well-being of its populace. Nonetheless, it was two centuries later that transboundary cooperation to prevent the spread of diseases received significant attention. Albeit this appeared more closely associated with economies, commerce, and travel than health concerns. Health became one of the first cross-border issues to engage in multilateral diplomatic tactics in the 19th century.[9]

The *Conseil Superieur de la Sante* (Superior Council of Health) of Constantinople was established in 1838 to oversee sanitation at the Turkish ports and prevent the spread of cholera. This council, which comprised of delegates from the Ottoman Empire and the chief maritime states, led to the first international health organization, the *Office Internationale d'Hygiène Publique* (Office of International Public Hygiene). The purpose was to monitor and exchange information to protect against the spread of infectious diseases. This cooperation became the foundation for the International Sanitary Conferences of the 1850s, and one of the earliest indicators of health diplomacy. Some scholars suggest this was likely motivated by a priority to prevent the spread of infectious diseases from the East to the West during maritime trade. Aginam opined that such international health diplomacy was based upon the European-dominated International Sanitary Conferences where he questioned such international relationship as more concerned about protecting the North from diseases of the South.[10] He further argues that it was the 19th-century power and hegemony that led to both international public health diplomacy and the health divide that exists today, where "[T]he colonial origins of public health diplomacy in the 19th Century, with its indelible fingerprints on polarisation of society according to the standards of civilisation, has continued to shape and re-shape the contours of global health governance."[11] David Fidler identified the first 100 years of health diplomacy (1851–1951) as the response to the concern of transboundary diseases.[12] Diplomatic approaches became necessary since "[C]onflicts frequently arose as nations sought to balance territorial sovereignty and economic interests with the need for transparent and universally applied health protections."[13]

The International Sanitation Conferences evolved as the origin of health diplomacy in the modern world, shaping new networks of collaboration across health professionals and decision-makers for the purpose of implementing policies to prevent transborder spread of diseases. While the shift in knowledge from contagion to germ theory progressed over the centuries, public health actions continued to prevent outbreaks. Scientists may not have known the actual causes of plague, cholera, and vector-borne diseases; however, these conferences established the essential networks for decision-makers and allied health fields to design and implement policies to control infectious diseases beyond one geographic or political border. With increased human interactions and maritime trade, more opportunities to be exposed to new germs were expected. Therefore, transborder cooperation and the promotion of health diplomacy became the cornerstone of preventing and monitoring the spread of diseases.

In the Americas, it was the Sanitary Conferences, first organized to respond to the threat of diseases and pestilences, which led to the Pan American Sanitation Bureau (PASB) in 1902 and known today as the Pan American Health Organization (PAHO). Regional health cooperation during this time focused on the deadly threats of cholera, plague, and yellow fever (YF). Also, the *Office Internationale d'Hygiène Publique* (Paris, 1906), the League of National Health Organization (Geneva, 1920), and the World Health Organization (WHO, 1948) all provided the foundation of organizations involved in the development of international health cooperation. A PAHO regional meeting was convened in Havana in 1924 to draft the first Pan American Sanitary Code. The purpose was to prevent the spread of diseases, promote cooperation for regional health issues, standardize data collection and disease protection methods, and improve upon ways to share health information in the region. The early collective actions, along with collaborative scientific research and policy coordination, became a priority to control YF and malaria in the Americas whereby regional scientific diplomacy enabled the successful construction of the Panama Canal when workers confronted persistent disease threats.

Article 54 of the Constitution of the WHO states that

> The Pan-American sanitary organization represented by the Pan-American Sanitary Bureau and the Pan-American Sanitary Conferences, and all other inter-governmental regional health organizations in existence prior to the date of signature of this Constitution, shall in due course be integrated with the Organization. This integration shall be effected as soon as practicable through common action based on mutual consent of the competent authorities expressed through the organizations concerned.[14]

It is important to re-emphasize that PAHO was well developed 46 years before the founding of the WHO in 1948; yet it wasn't until 1969 that the International Health Regulations (IHR), the regulatory arm of the WHO, was formalized during the 22nd World Health Assembly (WHA). Over the years the IHR was minimally modified until the deadly coronavirus, severe acute respiratory syndrome (SARS), was first identified in February 2003 in Asia. This compelled the WHO in 2005 to implement new criteria for reporting and disseminating information about a public health emergency of international concern (PHEIC). Prior to this event, IHR mandated disease outbreak reporting for YF, plague, and cholera in the 21st century, an outdated approach for preventing the spread of new and old diseases.

Case Study 5.1

Yellow Fever: Then and Now

YF is a mosquito-borne viral hemorrhagic disease that is endemic in parts of Central and South America still today with both sylvatic (jungle) and urban outbreaks enduring. It is transmitted by the *Aedes aegypti* mosquito that also causes dengue, chikungunya, and Zika virus, but there is only a vaccine for YF. Such vector-borne diseases present significant public health challenges in this hemisphere of which Zika virus has received the most attention recently.

In the early 1900s, collaborative research, diplomatic cooperation, and policy coordination between Cuba, Panama, and the United States buttressed the successful completion of the Panama Canal. It was the French who commenced the construction of the Panama Canal in 1881, and unable to fend off their stinging nemesis, the vectors of disease became victorious by 1888. It took science and vaccine diplomacy coupled with the wider contribution of diplomatic engagement to control the spread of YF. The importance of early transborder collaboration to control YF existed even when less sophisticated epidemiological techniques to track disease spread were available. Furthermore, the challenge to combat the deadly YF disease highlights how development, globalization, disasters, health diplomacy, and health security are all important to the disease then and now.

Background and History

YF arrived in the Americas by way of colonial slave trade from Africa.[15] Low levels of YF transmission were first identified in Yucatan in 1566. In 1648, travelers from Yucatan introduced this disease into Cuba where it waned until it was re-introduced by infected prisoners from Veracruz who were brought there in 1751 to build cabanas. The disease remained endemic in Cuba until 1901.[16] The collaboration between Cuba, Panama, and the United States identified YF as a virus in the early 1900s, and in 1915 a Yellow Fever Commission funded by the Rockefeller Foundation and led by virologist Max Theiler ultimately developed the YF vaccine by 1938. Research trials were held in Brazil that year showing great success and eventually earning Theiler the Nobel Prize in Medicine in 1951. This demonstrates the early value of scientific and vaccine diplomacy.

The 19th-century health officials used quarantine more for economic than health concerns.[17] Then in 1902 the PASB commenced a regional effort to control the spread of YF and share information, serving as a new model for transborder regional cooperation in health. The construction of the Panama Canal, which began in 1881, most likely would not have come to fruition without the public health cooperation between Cuba, Panama, and the United States. Merciless mosquitoes carrying YF and malaria devastated the French workers forcing them to abandon their labors to build the canal in 1888. The battle against YF was finally controlled in Cuba through the work of Carlos Finlay, a distinguished Cuban medical doctor and less-known US Army physician and Surgeon General, George Miller Sternberg, along with Walter Reed a U.S. Army physician and William Gorgas, Chief Sanitary Officer in Havana.[18] Targeting mosquito-breeding sites, promoting good sanitation practices, and implementing quarantine methods previously used for cholera spirited a new era of regional cooperation for public health research and practices.

The United States took control to build the canal in 1904 and maintained the Canal Zone until President Jimmy Carter signed the Panama Canal Treaty on September 7, 1977 transferring ownership to Panama before 2000. For the past 20 years, Panama has maintained ownership and in 2016 a $5 billion project expanded the canal to accommodate larger containerships for increased trade.

Yellow Fever Today

Even though there is an effective vaccine with long time protection, outbreaks continue because of low immunization coverage. According to WHO, the habitat of the *Aedes aegypti* mosquito has spread to both rural and urban areas and currently YF is endemic in ten countries in Latin America and several more in the Caribbean. Populations remain disproportionately impacted with loggers and miners working in the forest at greatest risk of the sylvatic YF transmission. Urban outbreaks are at the highest rates in 50 years.[19]

In 2008, an urban YF outbreak in "Paraguay was able to implement a timely and rapid vaccination response. Before the arrival of vaccines, civil disturbance was mounting in the face of public panic."[20] Paraguay had limited supply of YF vaccine, so neighboring countries mobilized their resources to ensure 3.5 million vaccines reached the country. This exemplifies diplomacy to promote regional good will, humanitarianism, and national interests to control the outbreak within Paraguay.[21]

Increased local urban transmission in Brazil, coupled with vaccine shortages in 2016, created new challenges especially for the poor, where exposures to poor drainage created ideal environmental conditions for mosquito-breeding sites. This impacted the *favelas* (shanty towns) where the poor also had limited access to YF immunization. The Brazilian government, thinking that they had YF under control, sent millions of doses of the vaccine to Angola. This left the country without enough vaccines to meet their own population demands during this widespread outbreak. The United States also reported YF vaccine shortages. One approach, sensationalized through social media, portrays how a Brazilian drug leader kidnapped two nurses and vaccination supplies and brought them to one of the poorest communities in southeast Brazil, *Salgueiro favela*, to vaccinate residents against YF. Social media did not condemn these actions; rather, the drug lord was recognized as a modern-day Robin Hood.[22] The vaccinators were released unharmed; however, this raises an important question. Are vaccines a public good with equitable distribution for all? This is a timely discussion as the world watches the development, authorization, and ultimately the distribution of a COVID-19 vaccine.

Conclusion

Since 2016, the Centers for Disease Control and Prevention (CDC) announced that YF cases, among unvaccinated travelers to Latin America, have risen due to more of these local urban outbreaks. The re-emergence of YF associated with the development, globalization, climate change, and disasters is all important to understand the vector's wider relationship to public health and where diplomacy and security are well situated to carry out an effective response. In 2018, Brazil identified 1,900 cases of YF with 590 deaths. By 2019, the WHO declared a 24% case fatality rate from YF. According to the PAHO, just because a country doesn't require vaccination to enter the country, the risk from periodic local transmission of YF is an important factor in the decision to be immunized. In fact, YF is the only disease WHO/IHR require travelers to show the documentation of vaccination whenever entering countries with such regulations.[23]

I remember traveling to countries where local transmission occurs, and no one asks for the yellow card to verify immunization against YF as an important public health prevention strategy. There was no oversight or enforcement of vaccine requirements applied. Who would enforce this? Is it the responsibility of airlines, or national governments with entrance and exist considerations? We observe current efforts underway to screen and detect international travelers during the coronavirus pandemic and some suggest health verification cards or health passports may become necessary to manage international travel and reduce the spread of coronavirus. Will this extend beyond the current pandemic and apply to other infectious diseases of international concern? These are important questions to address for the future of health diplomacy in world affairs and a willingness of countries to cooperate when the economic priorities may supersede the health restrictions.

Contemporary Health Diplomacy Responses

Regional efforts to make HIV/AIDS lifesaving drugs accessible exemplify the power of negotiations. The 2001 World Trade Organization's Ministerial Conference in Doha, Qatar focused on reducing trade barriers with increasing global trade and reducing conflicts about intellectual property rights and the pharmaceutical industry. The strategies set forth were designed to improve the access to essential drugs and seek health equity for poor countries. Brazil's Ministry of Foreign Affairs, Ministry of External Affairs, along with the Minister of Health's public health leadership for evidence-based research, presented a diplomatic response. They sought the ability to create compulsory licenses that would allow Brazil to manufacture less costly HIV/AIDS drugs still under patent, circumventing the 20-year patent under the Trade-Related Intellectual Property Rights (TRIPS). The Doha round addressed the inequity issues to ensure lives would be saved, creating new norms in international trade agreements.

The WHA Resolution (WHA 61.21) shows the extension of such diplomacy when it adopted a global strategy to bridge public health, innovation, and intellectual property along with added revisions in WHA 62.15 that targets actions to alleviate the burden of diseases that disproportionately impact poor populations.[24] The WHO supported a creative way to innovate, build capacity, improve access to medicines, and mobilize resources by supporting a needs-driven approach rather than a market-driven research agenda, which would be beneficial to resource poor countries.[25]

Furthermore, Brazil's international negations on tobacco policies demonstrate the significance where national-level leadership is necessary for global health governance. The Oswaldo Foundation in Brazil has taken a regional leadership role to address global health diplomacy with special attention to the South-South collaborations.[26] Since 1984, the *Tratado de Paz y Amistad* (Treaty of Peace and Friendship) between Chile and Argentina was introduced to affirm a joint commitment to strengthen their cross-border relationships. Both countries have continued to do "so" through important social, economic, and health collaborative initiatives.[27] This underscores how the convergence of domestic and international issues places public health into the wider foreign policy agenda where formal diplomacy is essential, while the rise in multistakeholder and multilateral informal diplomacy creates opportunities to better understand competing interests. Studying global and regional public health challenges such as HIV/AIDS, tobacco consumption, and pandemics further elucidates the inextricable relationship of economics to national and foreign policy interests[28] while emphasizing the many levels of health diplomacy.

Health as a Bridge to Peace

Contemporary health diplomacy made its mark in 1981 when the WHA Resolution 34.38[29] proposed that the function of health workers is to preserve and promote peace as a necessary path to achieve health for all.

In the Americas, health diplomacy was realized in 1984 during the U.S. backed "Contra" war in Central America when the PAHO coined the term Health as a Bridge to Peace (HBP). According to the WHO, HBP is defined as "the integration of peace-building concerns, concepts, principles, strategies and practices into health relief and health sector development," so that health can "transcend political, economic, social, and ethnic divisions among people and between nations"[30] and foster greater dialogue across combatants within and across countries. The intent was to apply a multidimensional approach to peace building that could improve public health, promote peace, and facilitate the delivery of health programs in times of civil conflict.[31] This is a reminder that the principles of the WHO were always based on "the health of all peoples is fundamental to the attainment of peace and security and is dependent upon the fullest co-operation of individuals."[32]

Through this HBP initiative, the PAHO proposed a polio immunization plan with greater cooperation and negotiation strategies between the El Salvadorian government and the *Frente Farabundo Martí para la Liberación Nacional* (FMLN, Farabundo Martí National Liberation Front) insurgent fighters, ultimately bringing together other non-state actors. Combatants agreed to put down their weapons and respect Days of Tranquility in order to immunize children. This joint polio campaign cultivated opportunities for greater dialogue, leading to new agreements and the support of other childhood vaccination programs. According to the PAHO, with the agreement of a cease fire, more than 20,000 health workers, volunteers, and opposition forces all worked together to immunize 250,000 children against childhood diseases throughout El Salvador. The cooperation from the government, rebels, PAHO, UNICEF, International Red Cross, religious groups, and Rotary Club made this possible with yearly designated Days of Tranquility beginning from 1985 to 1991. This concept of building peace through health caught on internationally with the WHO and the wider role of the United Nations in how preventive diplomacy through health could be effective. In May 1998, the WHA officially adopted the HBP as part of the Health for All strategy for the new millennium.

Once conflict breaks out, health diplomacy shifts from primary prevention to a more secondary level of "preventing and minimizing the health and environmental consequences of war."[33] I am reminded of an experience in Honduras during the mid-1980s. We were visiting the area and saw an overburdened, under-supported hospital where young children slept, two children to a crib. This occurred while the U.S. government provided economic and military aid to the anti-Sandinistas, "Contras," who fought against the *Frente Sandinista de Liberación Nacional* (Sandinista National Liberation Front) in Nicaragua led by Marxists-Leninist President José Daniel Ortega Saavedra.[34] The border threats to Honduras exposed how some were forced to flee violence and the repression, presenting the human face of food insecurity. Health workers said that one of the young boys was suffering from protein calorie malnutrition and pellagra, a disease known for its 3D's of diarrhea, dementia, and dermatitis that makes the skin peel like flakes of paint. The fourth D is death. Pellagra was rare in this Central American nation since flour enriched with vitamin B3 (niacin) was widely available through consuming tortillas. We were given permission to reach out to the boy's mother. I was especially interested in talking with her when health workers said, "ellas esta un poco loca" (she is a little crazy), since she believed evil spirits in the ground caused her son to become gravely ill. I asked her to explain why she thought her son was sick, and it was no surprise that the mother's perception of evilness was substantiated by the upheaval of her small plot of land, possibly due to landmines, and their inability to farm the land any longer. The land was infiltrated by something evil.

This was another reminder that listening to why people think they get sick helps to explain the underlying factors that contribute to the instability of health, safety, and security of peoples. She was not crazy. Not ignorant. She understood the evilness that was bestowed upon her precious plot of land caus- ing her and her family to flee for fertile lands that would keep them safe. Upon our return visit a few days later, the mother was gone and shortly after the child passed. I remember that incident clearly since it taught me about asking many questions and not only listening to the "experts." Not that the medical doctors could have saved the frail child as he reached the hospital too late, but it is a re- minder to respect a mother's understanding of tragic situation by just listening to her stories. His death was another entry into the database. And still, the root causes are situated within the social, political, economic, and environmental determinants of health.

Six years later, I was getting ready to give a talk about public-private part- nerships at the Pan American Development Foundation Conference in the af- termath of Hurricane Andrew (1992) in South Florida, but I was caught off guard. I was told the projector was not working and I could not use my pre- pared carrousel of slides for the presentation. It was 1992 and this was the go-to method for talks before the availability of Power Point, Google slides, or Adobe programs of today. It would be a large assembly, and what could I talk about to engage the audience if I did not use charts, graphs, or pictures? A well-experienced first responder colleague was with me, and I recalled that he recently asked me, "why do you ask so many questions?" This was followed by "You're like my five-year daughter." Was this a compliment or a criticism?

I proceeded to use his question and statement, and I began with, "Children are expected to ask a lot of questions, but adults are not." When adults ask too many questions, we are considered to be impolite, or ill-informed with the ex- pectation that one should already know the answers. Asking questions provides a more in-depth level of awareness about the different perceptions of a situa- tion. I thought back to my experience with that caring, not so crazy mother of the dying young boy in the crib. In order to engage people with one another we need to find a way to facilitate cooperation and create a synergy for a more robust collaboration and one that respects a mother's perception. Different governmental and nongovernmental groups working together to improve community-based health, safety, or security may all have the same goal in mind, while their objectives and strategies may actually collide rather than cooperate. This arises when privacy or state security issues may impede cooperation across the different stakeholders and could likely exacerbate the lack of trust people have with their government, agencies, or organizations. It starts by taking the time to listen to the different voices and not disregard the competing perspectives on the issues which brought them to the confrontation.

Identifying ways to cooperate is not necessarily an easy path. However, public health diplomacy actions, through Days of Tranquility or by creating more formal truces to immunize children, have been well documented in El Salvador from 1985 to 1991. Other terms, such as Corridors of Peace or Zone of Peace, continue to be used throughout the world today. And yes, diplomacy is as much about negotiation with governments, nongovernmental organizations, public-private partnerships or others, as it is about listening. This applies to perceptions and perspectives on public health as much as it does about implementing other national or foreign policies. This is where vaccine diplomacy crisscrosses international relations, public health, and science.

Vaccine Diplomacy

No human disease other than smallpox has been eradicated. Smallpox eradication was possible due to the availability and accessibility of vaccines and the impressive global commitment and cooperation to immunize individuals. The term vaccine diplomacy is part of the wider global public health diplomacy approach for equitable access to vaccines across rich and poor countries. Dr. Peter Hotez uses the term vaccine science diplomacy to emphasize the informal role of scientist-to-scientist collaborations to develop both lifesaving vaccines and related technologies.[35] Using Katz et al.'s three levels of diplomacy discussed previously, vaccine diplomacy exemplifies the shifts from the traditional nation-nation diplomacy to multistakeholders such as the UNICEF and the Global Alliance of Vaccine (Gavi), as well as more informal levels between scientist-to-scientist and private foundations.

Vaccines and transborder diplomacy from the 19th-century scientific collaborations of Englishman Edward Jenner's smallpox vaccine, French Louis Pasteur's rabies vaccine in the late 1880s, to U.S. Albert Sabin's polio vaccine in the 20th century show the important intersection of vaccines and diplomacy.[36] Scientific cooperation and vaccine collaboration have been key factors in improving population health outcomes; however, it is the refusal to cooperate that may stand out as more notable in bringing attention to the global inequities and mutual benefit from vaccines. An example of a lack of collaboration occurred in December 2006 when the Indonesia Minister of Health, Siti Fadilah Supari, refused to share H5N1influenza (bird flu) viral samples with the WHO. Supari argued that Indonesia owned the rights to viruses circulating within their country. She recognized such rights under the 1992 treaty signed at the United Nations Convention of Biological Diversity giving countries fair and equitable benefits from sharing viral strains. Calling for viral sovereignty, Supari contended that the Global South would not benefit equally from vaccine development in the Global North, since their flu samples were to be used to patent vaccines disproportionately available and accessible to the rich countries who could afford to purchase them. Negotiations took years and drew attention to inequities in access to vaccines.[37] Dr. David Heiman, head of infectious diseases at the WHO, "thanked Indonesia for drawing attention to the problem and said he had assured that it would not hold the W.H.O. hostage to the virus."[38] Holbrooke and Garrett contested that claiming viral sovereignty is "morally reprehensible," since influenza strains "can be carried across international borders by migratory birds[39] and cause much greater risks.

As previously described in Chapter 3, globalization's increased transborder risks require greater transparency in sharing timely information to prevent outbreaks and potential pandemics. While WHO's multilateral diplomacy struggled to foster cooperation in Indonesia, it was the more informal role of science-to-science collaboration to get Indonesia to provide their viral strains[40] and eventually share their human virus samples circulating within the country. After years of international negotiations, in April 2011 the WHO established the Pandemic Influenza Preparedness (PIP) Framework which changed the sharing of viral strains and the benefit sharing system for a more equitable access to influenza vaccines in resource poor countries.[41]

The history of regional cooperation for YF vaccine to more current approaches to equitable access emphasizes the demand for broader collaborative efforts to procure vaccines and related supplies. In 1977, PAHOs Revolving Fund became a model for other regions of the world with pooling resources, obtaining high-quality vaccines, and maintaining lower costs. This regional success ensured people would be vaccinated against diseases such as measles, polio, and YF and more based upon the principles of equity, solidarity, and economies of scale.[42] This exemplifies regional governance and readiness for immunization, cold chain, and supply chain demands. It also recognized the significance of the interrelationship of public health and economics, reinforcing an understanding that increasing access to vaccinations will protect both the economy and public health. The collaborative efforts from scientific discoveries and vaccine development to the distribution, equitable access, and compliance to immunize populations will be tested in 2021 with the SARS-COV-2 vaccines. This is where diplomacy on behalf of international relations and science aimed at public health co-exist, with a wider respect for the social, cultural, political, economic, environmental, and technological factors essential to successful outcomes.

Chagas Disease: Regional Health Diplomacy

Latin America's cooperation to battle Chagas disease is another excellent example of regional diplomacy. This came to fruition in the 1990s because Chagas disease was identified as the top parasitic infection in Latin America with enormous social and economic impact, and limited discussion beyond the medical and public health literature. It is also known as *American trypanosomiasis*, which is different than the better-known *African trypanosomiasis*, sleeping sickness. More people seem to be aware of the tsetse fly that causes sleeping sickness in Africa than the odd looking triatomine bug that causes both acute and chronic conditions in the Americas. Chagas disease is an important neglected tropical disease and one of the most common "affecting the bottom 100 million in the region."[43] According to the CDC, an estimated 7 million people are infected in 26 countries throughout Mexico, Central and South America, as well as 300,000 cases in the United States. April 14, 2020, World Chagas Disease Day, was the first time the WHO recognized Chagas as a wider global health concern, with the increasing spread of the disease beyond Latin America into the United States, Canada, Europe, and parts of Western Pacific countries. The WHO estimates there are 10,000 deaths each year and 75 million people around the globe at risk.[44]

Background and History

Brazilian physician Carlos Chagas first discovered the disease in 1909, which was later determined to be caused by a parasite, *Trypanosoma cruzi*. It is transmitted by the reduviid bug that deposits infective feces into the skin when biting its human victim. It is also referred to as the kissing bug because of its nighttime activity to drop from the roofs to bite an unsuspecting target where the bug comfortably resides in crevices of poorly constructed homes. It can also be transmitted through infected blood products during transfusion, organ transplants, and from mother to child during birth.

The social and environmental determinants are important since the triatomine bug lives in poor housing often found in rural and peri-urban areas throughout Latin America. The contributing factors of population growth and urbanization in South America during the 1970s and 1980s changed the pattern of Chagas, bringing it into the cities. Rising temperatures have also accelerated the production of the vector, *t. cruzi*,[45] adding further challenges in responding to the prevention and control of Chagas disease.

In 2010, the Ecuadorian Ministry of Public Health reported 1.38% of the population tested positive for the parasite *t. cruzi* in their blood with approximately one in every 50 people infected by the *chinchorro* triatomine bug as it is referred to in Ecuador.[46] In 2013, it was reported that Chagas was endemic in 21 countries in Latin America, an incidence of 28,000 cases in the Americas, with 8 million people in Latin America infected. According to the WHO there were 12,000 cases in Colombia and 30,000 living with the *t. cruzi* in United States.[47]

Collaborative research on synthetic insecticides shows how scientific diplomacy began in 1940s and continued through the 1970s using synthetic pyrethroid insecticides, which were low cost, safe, and effective to control the vector. The first campaigns to control Chagas took place in Brazil in 1983.[48] This was followed by international surveillance and vector control efforts through the 1990s into early 2000.

Regional Cooperation

Chagas collaboration in the Southern Cone of South America had been well documented in the literature,[49] where the first regional agreements for Chagas took place in 1991 known as the Southern Cone Initiative to Control/Eliminate Chagas (INCOSUR). This included seven countries in South America: Argentina, Bolivia, Brazil, Chile, Paraguay, Peru, and Uruguay with scientific support research groups in 22 countries. The INCOSUR Collaboration highlights regional cooperation along with cost-effective interventions for public health. Each nation maintained the responsibility for financing and managing of the project within their countries with collective technical and diplomatic cooperation and coordination. There are multiple reasons for this regional success including technical cooperation, regional economic growth and political will to invest in Chagas, and stable political systems with good regional diplomatic relationships.[50] The Southern Cone Collaborative Initiative (1991) was followed by the Andean Pact Initiative and the Central American Initiative both in 1997.

Successes showed how investments in public health produced economic returns motivating other countries to join together to tackle Chagas. Science and technology brought safe insecticide while the political will and economic investments made this possible. The PAHO provided the technical assistance to disseminating information and facilitating meetings. Uruguay's Minister of Health, Alfredo Solari, remarked "there has been a clear sense of joint responsibility and commitment by countries with common borders."[51] While respecting state sovereignty, the movements of populations across borders and rise in globalization helped to organize regional efforts against Chagas.

Case Study 5.2

Health Diplomacy – Negotiating Indigenous Health

Valdivia, Rivera et al. describe how Chile, Peru, and Bolivia collaborated to reduce conflict related to cross-border issues of Indigenous Peoples. Chile led the efforts to establish intercultural health, which embraces the respect for indigenous knowledge and health practices into public health practices.[52]

My initial experience with health diplomacy occurred in 1986, even though I may not have fully recognized this term at the time. It took place during a collaborative community-based participatory research project to control the spread of scabies with the Guna Indians, Panama. Located on the northeast coast of Panama, formerly known as the San Blas archipelago, today this territory is referred to by its indigenous name, Guna Yala. This semi-autonomous territory is home to more than 60,000 Indigenous People where 360 islands exist, of which approximately 66 are inhabitable ranging from small to large island and mainland communities. Guna territory received its independence from Panama during the *Tule* (people) Revolution in 1925 and since has maintained its control with support from the Panamanian government as requested and accepted. Historically, Guna society has been recognized for their leadership and governance, documented and elucidated in the extensive research conducted over many decades by the distinguished anthropologist James Howe.[53]

Scabies, an ectoparasitic disease, is caused by a tiny mite that borrows under the skin presenting intense itching, disrupting sleep, study, or work routines and can lead to secondary bacterial infection. It's a global public health problem often seen in overcrowded living arrangements and where there is a lack of reliable access to potable water, such as among internally displaced populations and refugee settings. Scabies was new to the Guna communities, arriving sometime between 1972 and 1973 and rapidly spread across the villages by 1976. The University of Miami's Field Epidemiology Survey Team (FEST), in collaboration with the Panamanian Ministry of Health and local communities, began community research on scabies shortly after its arrival in the 1970s. This research recognized that treating only clinically identified cases of scabies, without responding to the wider community epidemiology, was "unlikely to have a significant impact in epidemic situations."[54] Therefore, a wider community-based approach was suggested as a more effective way to manage scabies within a community.

Public Health Diplomacy – Community-Based Program for Scabies

David Taplin, head of the FEST, and I arrived by *cayuco*, a dugout canoe, buoyed by a small horsepower engine to land on the island of Ticantiki/ Niadub. Upon arrival in 1986, we were ushered into the *congreso* (community gathering house) to explain our presence. We shared the letters of reference from both the Ministry of Health and more importantly from other Guna *sahilas* (chiefs) in nearby communities where we were working. We presented an appeal to respond to the growing concern of scabies in their community. Leaders and community members listened carefully as we suggested an innovative public health approach with the necessary teamwork from local to national leaders, traditional and Western health practitioners, and all community participants. This would require full cooperation across the community and beyond with outside partnerships including the pharmaceutical industry, and academia, and *Ministerio de Salud Panama (MINSA*, Ministry of Health Panama).

There was great interest since scabies was widespread with no answer to mitigate its spread. By the 1980s, Panama showed some resistance to the commonly used scabicide treatment known as Lindane. We knew that the challenge to implement a community- wide approach would require close collaboration, cooperation, communication, and culturally appropriate strategies

First, we gained the permission and support of the *sahilas* to open a field station where we could take up residence on the island. Garnering their political will was the first step. Second, we secured the assistance of the traditional health providers since they had no effective treatment to the scabies epidemic. They applied *Genipa americana*, black saptur, to cover the body, but it would not kill the tiny mite. Consequently, the respected traditional healers were eager to collaborate and some even stepped up early to receive treatment of a safe permethrin-based cream. Permethrin is derived from the chrysanthemum flower family and was shown to be an efficient, efficacious, and safe treatment for scabies. None of this could have been possible without a well-funded research grant from Burroughs Wellcome Company, USA and later the Welcome Foundation support. We collaborated with local and national community health workers supported by the Ministry of Health to identify best practices to inform, educate, and engage the community starting with a prevalence survey of rates of infestation on the island. Collaboratively we created the acronym, *Eliminacion de Escabiosis* Niadub (EDEN) (elimination of scabies in Niadub)[55] as the campaign. Lastly, with input from the community and a local health committee review panel, along with the approval from the university's Institutional Review Board and the Panamanian ministry of health, we designed this collective community-based scabies elimination program. A robust community-based program was necessary since 33% of the total population of 756 had active scabies.[56] The island was surveyed using a single engine aircraft and a map that would help identify each residence, whether it was made of cane and thatched roof or a cement building. The community was divided into four colors representing blue, green, red, and yellow sectors. The local health committee selected four women to serve their sectors and conduct house-to-house demographic surveys. Each sector leader was responsible for approximately 200 people, an estimated 25 families, where they selected four additional assistants in their sector. Training on the identification of scabies, collection of mites, applying topical treatment, ongoing communication and testing protocol, logistical and project management was possible since two members of the research team would always be on the island. All household members received their 5% permethrin cream treatments in the evening with follow-up in the morning to bathe and wash off the cream. The ongoing efforts to control scabies were made possible through negotiations with the *sahilas*. Community leaders made the decision for everyone to receive the topical treatment and added a policy that anyone leaving or arriving to the island would receive treatment. Paid local assistants continued to conduct surveillance, and scabies remained below 1.5% over three years.

As discussed throughout this book, public health matters do not happen in isolation to the wider national, regional, or global political and economic issues. The United States invasion of Panama in 1989[57] caused weeks of disruption and access to the supply of medication, and the prevalence of scabies crept up to 12% over three months.[58] Diplomacy broke down, and public health suffered. However, the control of scabies reduced the incidence of skin infections and use of antibiotics, and an unexpected outcome was the reduction in head lice, until it crawled back into the community after the community hosted a regional volleyball tournament.

The research supported that an outbreak of scabies in a community is best controlled by treating symptomatic individuals along with their contacts versus only treating individuals with active scabies. Scabies remains a public health challenge in many resource poor regions, and due to costs the community-based treatment approach is not sustainable. This presents an ethical dilemma in conducting research if benefits to the people are not sustainable. Such lessons were learned when research for HIV/AIDS, to determine seroprevalence rates in the world, generated many questions about identifying a disease without providing treatment. This compelled researchers to ensure that the continual access to HIV/AIDS lifesaving drugs was available, accessible, and utilized. Unfortunately, this was not the case with scabies.

Discussion

Learning new information is a two-way process. While Ticantiki/Niadub did not have microscopes to identify the mite, women used a safety pin to puncture the skin to remove the microscopic mite. Safety pins were plentiful since they were the only way to hold up baby's diapers.

The art and science of removing the microscopic scabies mite or eggs amazed me in how ingenious the Guna women were. This was the first of many lessons offered, and where the most valuable public health education often takes place.

Ticantiki/Niadub had a community health post with limited facilities and no electricity. The health center was led by a local health auxiliary nurse, Juana Herrera, who was trained in Panama City and returned to her community. She did everything from vaccinations, well care, to delivery of babies. She was supported by a community health worker, a medical records data manager, and a *cayuco* motorist who would travel with her and patients that needed transport to one of the larger islands for more treatment options. FEST, led by the forward thinking of Taplin, fitted out this health post with the first-ever solar energy health center in the region. Juana no longer had to use a kerosene lantern to deliver a baby in the middle of night. The 1986 solar panels remained active for decades until the battery stopped working and ultimately was replaced by the Ministry of Health with a newer version more than 20 years later.

In the 1980s, Guna population considered their health a private matter and would welcome a traditional healer into their home before going to the Westernized health care center. We observed while working in other communities that indigenous populations did not always trust the Panamanian health providers, and there were few Guna providers. Therefore, from the scabies assessments to treatments to follow up efforts took place from house to house, using traditional music and dance to engage the interest and fit with the culturally accepted norms of the general population. Notwithstanding, a Guna medical doctor served as the Ministry of Health's Regional Director during the time of this research program. Currently there are more Guna nurses, nutritionists, and physicians meeting community health needs with cultural competency of indigenous practices and wider acceptance of Western health and medical practices.

The Cuban government provided a welcomed opportunity to train Guna students as future doctors through a cooperative agreement with Panama. In early 2000, there were about 40 or more students selected by the Guna General Congress to study medicine in Cuba with the intent for them to return to Panama and work in their communities. I know a few Guna medical doctors that received full scholarships to study at Cuba's *Escuela Latino Americana de Medicina* (ELAM) (Latin American School of Medicine) where they spent two years in Havana followed by four years in the provinces. Their studies and practical training prepared them well, and they have become valued health providers within their communities.

Conclusion

The foundation of the EDEN scabies program rested upon science, technology, public health activities, diplomacy, and creating partnerships. The value of diplomacy in public health events became an important lesson learnt. Encouraging reciprocal respect across different actors at all levels, taking the time to understand local governance and elder leadership, acquiring patience and more listening skills, and building relationships across the many partnerships were the necessary underlying factors to optimize diplomacy as a bridge for public health.

Transborder Data Sharing of Public Health

Countries continue to willfully withhold releasing timely data about a disease outbreak. The clear objective of transborder health cooperation simply ceases to exist without the early sharing of information. China has long been criticized for such actions; however, we can look closer to home with the Zika outbreak and Venezuela's lack of transparency as well as dengue and cholera in Cuba. The decision to forsake timely sharing of data on disease outbreak at home raise important local to regional to global health governance issues. This is an unmistakable reminder that the controversial purpose of the International Sanitary Conference to protect economic health over public health continues to challenge effective responses.

Case Study 5.3

A Paradox in Public Health Diplomacy U.S.–Cuba Relationship[59]

Before the 2010 earthquake devasted Haiti and a deadly cholera outbreak spread to other Caribbean nations, in 1991 cholera first re-emerged in this hemisphere after a 100-year absence. The El Tor strain of *Vibrio cholera* arrived in Peru via a Chinese cargo ship along the coast of Peru just north of the capital city, Lima. According to the PAHO from 1991 to 1997 cholera affected 21 countries in the region with 1.2 million cases and almost 12,000 deaths. The epidemic spread through South America into Central America and Mexico.[60]

As discussed earlier, cholera stirred conspicuous fear in the 19th century, prompting the first, of many, International Sanitation Conferences to prevent and control the spread of disease. Even then, and not knowing what caused cholera, countries agreed to cooperate and share health information as a way to reduce the extent of cholera. Today, accelerated migration, trade, travel, tourism, disasters, and climate change underscore the spatial and temporal dimensions to explain a more rapid disease spread. Albeit, now we have improved epidemiology and public health preparation coupled with remarkable advances in scientific and mass media tools to respond to cross-border health threats such as cholera and dengue. Even with such advancements, there remains a continuing debate if the impetus for these early international meetings was fueled by the fear of disrupting trade and commerce versus the protection of population health. Consequently, with advanced knowledge, and home to the world-recognized Pedro Kourí Institute of Tropical Medicine founded in 1937, we have to question whether the Cuban government prioritizes their need for tourism dollars more than local public health demands? To understand more recent infectious disease outbreaks in Cuba, it is instructive to explore the inextricable relationship of three factors: increase of globalization, travel, and tourism; lack of government transparency, highlighted by the palpable dishonesty of past and current infectious disease outbreaks; and the decline of their public health infrastructure as mentioned in previous chapters.[61]

The spread of water-borne (e.g. cholera) and vector-borne (e.g. dengue) diseases is central to the discussion of globalization where trade, business travel, and tourism expose the reality that infectious diseases do not respect borders. The life-threatening microbes and vectors of disease cross borders freely without any documentation of their existence, until they become the unwelcomed visitors. In 2010, Cuba was listed as 9th for the most international tourist arrivals in the Americas reporting a 7% increase for that year.[62] Consequently, the loss of tourism and trade currency presents a clear threat to the health of the Cuban economy.

History Re-Emergence of Mosquito-Borne Diseases

As seen above, the re-emergence of the *Aedes aegypti* mosquito has hit Latin America and the Caribbean especially hard with outbreaks of YF. Dengue is also transmitted by this mosquito; however, there is no vaccine available. Dengue and the life-threatening form called dengue hemorrhagic fever (DHF) has become the most serious mosquito-borne viral disease today.[63] This same mosquito also transmits chikungunya and Zika virus. Key issues such as globalization, urbanization, climate change, and natural disasters are some of the contributing factors of re-emerging of dengue and dengue hemorrhagic fever (D/DHF) with an estimated cost of US$ 2.1 billion a year.[64]

Dengue was first recorded in Cuba in the late 1820s and followed by the pandemic of 1850.[65] Outbreaks have continued in Cuba from the 1970s, 1980s–1990s, earlier denied, and again more recently. In 1981, Cuba faced the more life-threatening form of DHF epidemic killing 158 people of which 101 were children.[66]

Cuba has made significant scientific contributions regarding D/DHF for other countries to follow.[67] The concern is not about their scientific knowledge. It is more about Cuba's official reporting. In late August 2012, a dissident journalist reported that there were 400 cases of dengue in Camaguey while the government remained silent.[68] We also know more than a decade ago when health professionals were forbidden to use the words "dengue fever" since the Cuban government maintained an official position that the virus had been eradicated within Cuba's borders.

Dengue and Dengue Hemorrhagic Fever to Zika Virus

Dengue re-emerged in the Americas and in 1981 with the first epidemic of DHF in Cuba. The Cuban government implemented an active surveillance and mosquito control program and soon reported that they eliminated the disease while other countries struggled. Furthermore, reports of dengue surveillance revealed increasing spread throughout this hemisphere. In 1996, a confidential report from the Cuban government to *Médecins San Frontiers* (Doctors without Borders) discovered a request for 180 tons of insecticide and equipment to fight against the *A. aegypti* mosquitos that cause dengue.[69]

The deceptive decision to deny the existence of D/DHF generated world attention on June 25, 1977 when Dr. Dessy Mendoza Rivero, *Presidente de Colegio Médico Independiente de Santiago* (President of the Independent Medical College of Santiago), was arrested and charged with violating Cuba's Penal Code for disseminating "enemy propaganda" during a Radio Martí Miami radio interview where he documented 30,000 cases of dengue, 2,500 hospitalized, and 13 deaths including children all probably related to DHF. He was arrested at his home in Santiago de Cuba where the dengue outbreak struck hardest. On August 18, 1997, Amnesty International called him a prisoner of conscience, and on November 18, 1997 he was found guilty of spreading "enemy propaganda" and sentenced to eight years in prison. The Cuban government acknowledged the outbreak shortly after; however, even with international pressure it took 18 months for him to be released from the Boniato maximum security jail where he went into exile in Spain.[70] Sadly, today the situation does not appear to be much different.[71]

In an increasingly borderless world, with greater speed, further reach, and quicker exchange of people and cargos, both old and new diseases have gone global. Unlike the restriction of other undesirables there is no wall to prevent migrating mosquitoes from freely traveling. As a result, the rise in mosquito-borne diseases such as the Zika virus – along with dengue and chikungunya viral infections – has spread rapidly throughout the Americas. The main culprit is the highly resilient *A. aegypti* mosquito that has skillfully adapted to environmental and climate changes.

According to the PAHO, 22 countries and territories in the Americas reported transmission of the Zika virus since the first locally acquired cases were confirmed in Brazil in May 2015. Cuba, however, remained silent. Cuba's year (2015) of unprecedented drought, impact of natural disasters, and failing infrastructure of deteriorating water, sewage, and housing systems forms a perfect storm for the reality of a mosquito population explosion. This was especially significant since the *A. aegypti* mosquito, which can also transmit YF, dengue, chikungunya, and Zika virus, resides in Cuba with ongoing dengue transmission. In January 28, 2015, Haiti and Dominican Republic reported local transmission of the Zika virus, suggesting it is likely reached Cuba. Although Cuba reported no cases of chikungunya which seems highly unlikely since according to the PAHO statistics, all countries and territories in the Hispanic Caribbean, other Caribbean, in additional to Central and most South American countries and the United States have reported imported and local transmission occurrences since late 2013.[72]

In my interviews with people who traveled to communities in Cuba in November 2015, they shared stories of both dengue and cholera in the Santiago de Cuba province, which were well beyond the officially reported cases in the Holguín region. Cuba conducts very active surveillance with proactive community strategies to reduce the mosquito population and promote improved hygiene. Nevertheless, when someone becomes ill with dengue or cholera, the Cuban government uses euphemistic terms such as a febrile illness or gastrointestinal upset, which is concerning since Cuba has a well-developed disease surveillance system with highly skilled health professionals. Cuba's practice of *el silencio de epidemiológico* (epidemiologic silence)[73] stifles diplomacy and creates a health security risk.

Cholera Denied

Cuba was spared when the virulent cholera *El tor* strain re-emerged in this hemisphere on the Peruvian coast (1991). Absent since 1880, cholera did re-emerge in Cuba in 2012. Possibly, it was Cuba's participation in a medical diplomacy mission that brought cholera home. However, water and sanitation services remain "outdated, obsolete, and insufficient to meet the growing national demand for safe drinking water and adequate sanitation services"[74] and according to the data used by Belt and Velazquez, the access to piped drinking water was reported as 65% for the national population, and sewerage services reaching only 38% of the population.[75]

Less than three weeks after three deaths from cholera were officially reported on July 3, 2012, Cuba announced there were no new cases of cholera. Subsequently new cases appeared. Whether the Cuban cholera epidemic is blamed on transborder transmission from Haiti during a post-disaster humanitarian mission, or because of in-country tropical storms, flooding, hurricane destruction, climate change, displacement, overcrowding, or economic crisis, the fact is that public health practice begins and ends with a sound infrastructure. In an interview with a Cuban physician who arrived in the United States two years prior, he emphasized that the Oriental region in Manzanillo, where the cholera deaths were reported, has a long history of inconsistent potable water. He commented that many residents use their bathtub as a reservoir to store clean water and claimed that the public health infrastructure in Cuba has not garnered the same political will as the medical investments for health facilities that support health tourism and biotechnology research.[76]

Conclusion

The Cuban government enjoys the symbolism of their health tourism and medical diplomacy as a measure of their commitment to local health, while doctors and journalists have been censored or jailed for sharing timely health information. Today, evidence suggests a clear paradox in Cuba's cloaked health diplomacy and yet the global community continues to romanticize Cuba's humanitarian efforts abroad.

Health diplomacy as part of the U.S.–Cuba future relationship would mean much more than collaborating on research for drug and vaccine development, since it would also require sharing timely information. In the meantime, governments may need to change policies on travel notices and seek out other sources for a more reliable rapid reporting to promote transparency about emerging and re-emerging diseases, which will also require creative cooperation and new perspectives on health diplomacy.

U.S.–Cuba Cooperation on Ebola: Disgrace or Diplomacy?[77]

The deadly Ebola virus demonstrated why international cooperation is both complicated and necessary. When the PAHO extended an invitation for the United States to participate in a 2014 hemispheric meeting on Ebola, the location and timing of the meeting became a point of contention to some Cuban American leaders in South Florida. U.S. House Representative Mario Diaz-Balart (R–FL) called the U.S. participation "a disgrace."

First, the Ebola Regional Technical Meeting prompted criticism because the United States sent a government representative to Havana. On October 29–30, 2014, with 34 countries in attendance, participants met to identify gaps in preparedness, discuss regional strategies, and expand training, resources, and risk communication. The White House sent Dr. Nelson Arboleda, then with the CDC Central America's Regional Director, to Cuba. Dr. Arboleda was the perfect choice, formerly a CDC Disease Detective, a global health leader, a Colombian-American who is knowledgeable about the events in Latin America.

Second, disapproval was voiced that the U.S. government's participation in the meeting held in Cuba took place during an expanded summit of the *Alianza Bolivariana para los Pueblos de Nuestra América* (ALBA) (Bolivarian Alliance for the Peoples of Our America), a regional organization formed to minimize U.S. hegemony in the region. The reality of establishing global health security by reducing the scourge of deadly diseases cannot always be conducted through traditional approaches in international relations. History reminds us of such efforts. As described earlier, the PAHO has played a key role in facilitating regional health diplomacy actions during conflict, and this requires finding other ways to cooperate, even though formal state- to state-level diplomacy does not exist.

Historical to Contemporary Health Diplomacy

In 1901, the PASB demonstrated the power of regional health cooperation during the deadly outbreaks of cholera, plague, YF, and malaria. We saw how the early collaborative scientific and epidemiologic research between Panama, the United States, and Cuba on YF was the dynamic factor for the successful completion of the Panama Canal. The U.S. and former Soviet Union's cooperation during the height of the Cold War placed ideological differences aside to jointly eradicate smallpox. The 1980s "Contra" War's impact in Central America and vaccination campaigns were designed to promote cooperation and foster greater negotiations between the insurgent fighters and governments, with such Days of Tranquility, or formal truces, documented in El Salvador from 1985 to 1991. We have seen throughout history that it takes both governmental and nongovernmental actors to participate in public health diplomacy. According to Adams, Novotny, and Leslie, the term global health diplomacy identifies political shifts to meet shared health goals by strengthening relationships to fulfill the resource gaps.[78]

For example, an effective diplomacy approach took place by bringing together local mayors from Israel, Jordan, and Palestine on the Island of Peace to explore border threats of water, environment, and public health in communities along the Jordan River Valley. This was convened by the formerly known Friends of the Earth Middle East founded by Gideon Bromberg and referred to today as Eco Peace Middle East. I was honored to serve as a facilitator for the public health component that took place during the first meeting on March 9, 2005, in collaboration with the University of Miami's The Sue and Leonard Miller Center for Contemporary Judaic Studies and Middle East Peace Studies. The strategy was to promote peace initiatives including nongovernmental actors, in collaboration with local leaders and universities from their respective countries. The site selected for this first of its kind meeting served as a reminder of the March 1997 tragic murders of schoolgirls gunned down by a mentally ill Jordanian soldier. Jordan's King Hussein reached out to heal Israeli-Arab conflict and designated this site as a hope for peace.

The celebrated scientific cooperation in research at the Sanford F. Kuvin Center for the Study of Infectious and Tropical Diseases at Hebrew University, Israel and Al-Quds University in Palestine is another example of coming together to wage war against deadly diseases without formal diplomatic relations.[79] Such regional cooperation shows the value of science and health diplomacy. Discussions took place not by country groupings but rather by participants focusing on similar issues impacting their communities from the North or South Jordan River Valley. Identifying, discussing, and navigating collaborative solutions to water, environment, and public health challenges create an upstream approach to diplomacy beyond the traditional mechanisms. This can be applied to similar efforts in transnational border conflicts in the Americas where new forms of cooperation can improve local levels to wider regional population well-being.

Conclusion

These examples are meant to show that it is not necessary to be "friends" to join forces and fight against plagues. We saw this with the eradication of smallpox during the Cold War. Sometimes it takes academic, scientific, and other non-state actors, such as the PAHO, nongovernmental organizations, business, and academic institutions to promote diplomacy. However, when this includes official governmental level, countries must acknowledge their collective responsibilities. Transborder coordination of activities and disclosing a country's health risk are necessary factors in preventing and controlling the spread of diseases, whether it is related to a communicable or noncommunicable disease. We know that without effective transparency, health diplomacy becomes an empty façade, and worse, global health security is seriously compromised. The lessons learned about health transparency, diplomacy, and cooperation through strengthening public-private partnerships deserve greater attention. This was emphasized from the start of the Health for All movement at Alma-Ata, Russia (today known as Almaty, Kazakhstan) in 1978 to the United Nations 2000–2015 Millennium Development Goals, and current 2015–2030 Sustainable Development Goals.

Concluding Remarks

Diplomacy and health marry two distinct fields of study, research, and practice. Therefore, it is important that students of history and international and regional studies gain a more in-depth understanding about the history of population health, safety, and security, while those studying global health become better informed about the history of a region where international relations and diplomacy have influenced public health outcomes. Nevertheless, recognizing the transdisciplinarity of diplomacy and health issues requires a balanced approach with the wider space for old and new actors and arrangements in foreign policy.

The coronavirus pandemic shows the intersection of diplomacy and public health as well as the interrelationship with development, globalization, disasters, and security. Furthermore, it features the characteristics of vaccine, science, and disaster diplomacy as more than academic exercises. Public health diplomacy must be part of the foreign policy toolkit, and not a postscript.

Notes

1 Harley Feldbaum and Joshua Michaud, "Health Diplomacy and the Enduring Relevance of Foreign Policy Interests," *PLoS Medicine* 7, no. 4 (2010), doi:10.1371/journal.pmed.1000226.

2 Ilona Kickbusch, Gaudenz Silberschmidt, and Paulo Buss, "Global Health Diplomacy: The Need for New Perspectives, Strategic Approaches and Skills in Global Health," *Bulletin of the World Health Organization* 85, no. 3 (2007): 230–232, doi:10.2471/BLT.06.039222.

3 Vincanne A. Adams, Thomas E. Novotny, and Hannah Leslie, "Global Health Diplomacy," *Medical Anthropology* 27, no. 4 (2008): 315–323, doi:10.1080/01459740802427067.

4 Rebecca Katz et al., "Defining Health Diplomacy: Changing Demands in the Era of Globalization," *Milbank Quarterly* 89, no. 3 (2011): 503–523, doi:10.1111/j.1468-0009.2011.00637.x.

5 Ilona Kickbusch et al., "Global Health Diplomacy."

6 Peter Gleijeses, "Cuba's First Venture in Africa: Algeria, 1961–1965," *Journal of Latin American Studies* 28, no. 1 (1996): 159–195.

7 Maria Werlau, "Cuba's Health-Care Diplomacy: The Business of Diplomacy," *World Affairs* 175, no. 6 (2013): 57–67.

8 Andrew Jack, "Cuba's Medical Diplomacy," *The Financial Times*, May 14, 2010.

9 Ilona Kickbusch and Margarita Ivanova, "The History and Evolution of Global Health Diplomacy," in *Global Health Diplomacy: Concepts, Issues, Actors, Instruments, Fora and Cases*, eds. Ilona Kickbusch et al. (New York: Springer, 2013), 11–26.

10 Obijiofor Aginam, "The Nineteenth Century Colonial Fingerprints on Public Health Diplomacy: A Postcolonial View," *Law, Social Justice & Global Development* 1 (2003): 1–12.

11 Ibid, 7.
12 David P. Fidler, "The Globalization of Public Health: The First 100 Years of International Health Diplomacy," *Bulletin of the World Health Organization* 79, no. 9 (2001): 843–849.
13 Alexandra M. Stern and Howard Markel, "International Efforts to Control Infectious Disease, 1851 to the Present," *Journal of American Medical Association* 292, no. 12 (2004): 1475, doi:10.1001/jama.292.12.1474.
14 World Health Organization Constitution, Article 54, http://www.ncbi.nlm.nih.gov/pmc/articles/PMC1625885/pdf/amjphnation00639-0074.pdf.
15 John R. Pierce and Jim Writer, *Yellow Jack: How Yellow Fever Ravaged America and Walter Reed Discovered Its Deadly Secrets* (Hoboken, NJ: John Wiley, 2005), 9.
16 Ibid, 14.
17 Ibid, 20.
18 Ibid.
19 World Health Organization, "Yellow Fever: A Current Threat," accessed December 2, 2020, https://www.who.int/csr/disease/yellowfev/impact1/en/). What happened was *Aedes aegypti* mosquito was transmitting the virus to humans (see Thomas P. Monath, "Yellow Fever Vaccines," *Expert Review of Vaccines* 4, no. 4 (2005): 689–693).
20 Jon Kim Andrus, et al., "Global Health Security and the International Health Regulations," *BMC Public Health* 10, no. Suppl 1 (2010): S2, http://www.biomedcentral.com/1471-2458/10/S1/S2.
21 Jon Kim Andrus, et al., "Yellow Fever and Health Diplomacy: International Efforts to Stop the Urban Yellow Fever Outbreak in Paraguay," in *Negotiating and Navigating Global Health: Case Studies in Global Health Diplomacy*, eds. Ellen Rosskam and Ilona Kickbusch (Singapore: World Scientific Publishing Company, 2011), 391–403.
22 Callum Patton, "Gang Boss who Kidnapped Nurses to Vaccinate the Poor Hailed as Modern-Day Robin Hood," *Newsweek*, February 16, 2018, https://www.newsweek.com/gang-boss-who-kidnapped-nurses-vaccinate-poor-hailed-modern-day-robin-hood-808675.
23 World Health Organization, "International Health Regulations (2005)," *Annexes 2, 6, and 7*, https://www.who.int/ihr/IHR_2005_en.pdf.
24 World Health Organization, *Global Strategy and Plan of Action on Public Health, Innovation, and Intellectual Property* (Geneva: WHO, 2011), https://www.who.int/phi/publications/Global_Strategy_Plan_Action.pdf.
25 See World Health Organization, Intergovernmental Working Group on Public Health, Innovation and Intellectual Property Rights, https://www.who.int/phi/igwg/en/; Margaret Chan, Jonas Gahr Støre, and Bernard Kouchner, "Foreign Policy and Global Health: Working Together Toward a Common Goals," *Bulletin of the World Health Organization* 86, no. 7 (2008): 498; and Kelley Lee and Adam Kamradt-Scott, "The Multiple Meanings of Global Health Governance: A call for Conceptual Clarity," *Globalization and Health* 10, no. 28 (2014): 5–10.
26 See the comprehensive collection of works and conceptual analyses edited by Paulo Marchiori Buss and Sebastián Tobar in *Health Diplomacy and Global Health: Latin American Perspectives* (Rio de Janeiro: Editora Fiocruz, 2017).
27 Jorge Ramírez, et al., "Chile's Role in Global Health Diplomacy: A Narrative Literature Review," *Globalization and Health* 14, no. 108 (2018), doi:10.1186/s12992-018-0428-8.
28 Joshua Michaud and Jennifer Kates, "Global Health Diplomacy: Advancing Foreign Policy and Global Health Interests," *Global Health Science Practice* 1, no. 1 (2013): 24–28.

29 World Health Organization, "Humanitarian Health Action: Health as a Bridge for Peace," accessed May 10, 2014, http://www.who.int/hac/techguidance/hbp/en/.

30 World Health Organization, "Humanitarian Health Action: Health as a Bridge for Peace: Report on the First World Health Organization Consultative Meeting" (Les Pensière, Annecy, October 30–31, 1997), https://www.who.int/hac/techguidance/hbp/strategies_/en/.

31 World Health Organization, "Humanitarian Health Action: Health as a Bridge for Peace."

32 WHO Constitution.

33 Barry Levy and Victor W. Sidel, *War and Public Health* (1997; 2nd ed., Oxford, UK: Oxford University Press, 2007), 389.

34 Contras is an abbreviated term for *contrarrevolución* or counter-revolution, rebel fighters against the Sandinista government (1979 through early 1990s).

35 Peter J. Hotez, "'Vaccine Diplomacy': Historical Perspectives and Future Directions," *PLOS Neglected Tropical Diseases* 8, no. 6 (2014), doi:10.1371/journal.pntd.0002808.

36 See historical milestones in vaccine diplomacy in Peter J. Hotez, "Vaccine Diplomacy."

37 Colin McInnes and Kelley Lee, *Global Health and International Relations* (Cambridge, UK: Polity Press, 2012), 162.

38 Donald McNeill, "Indonesia Offering Samples of Bird Flu for Vaccines," *The New York Times*, February 17, 2007.

39 Richard Holbrooke and Laurie Garrett, "'Sovereignty' That Risks Global Health," *The Washington Post*, August 10, 2007.

40 Ibid.

41 For a more detailed account go to Jeremy Youde, "Viral Sovereignty," *Globalization and Health* (Lanham, MD: Rowman and Littlefield, 2020), 113–135.

42 Pan American Health Organization, "Revolving Fund Immunization Toolkit," https://www.paho.org/immunization-toolkit/?page_id=25.

43 Peter J. Hotez, et al., "Chagas Disease: "The New HIV/AIDS of the Americas," *PLoS Neglected Tropical Diseases* 6, no. 5 (2012): e1498, doi:10.1371/journal.pntd.0001498.

44 World Health Organization, "World Chagas Disease Day: April 14, 2000," https://www.who.int/campaigns/world-chagas-disease-day/2020.

45 Susana N. Asin and Silvia Catalá, "Development of Trypanosoma Cruzi in Triatoma Infestans: Influence of Temperature and Blood Consumption," *Journal of Parasitology* 81, no. 1 (1995): 1–7.

46 Anis Rassi and José Antonio Marin-Neto, "Chagas Disease," *The Lancet* 375, no. 9723 (2010): 1388–1402.

47 CDC, and José Rodrigues Coura, "Chagas Disease: Control, Elimination and Eradication. Is it possible?", *Memórias do Instituto Oswaldo Cruz* 108, no. 8 (2013), doi:10.1590/0074-0276130565.

48 Joao Carlos Pinto Dias, Antonio Carlos Silveira, and Chris J. Schofield, "The Impact of Chagas Disease Control in Latin America: A Review,"*Memórias do Instituto Oswaldo Cruz* 97, no. 5 (2002): 603–612, and Joao Carlos Pinto Dias, and Chris J. Schofield, "The Evolution of Chagas Disease (American trypanosomiasis) Control after 90 Years since Carlos Chagas Discovery," *Memórias do Instituto Oswaldo Cruz* 94 (1999): 103–121.

49 Ruth Levine, "Case 12: Controlling Chagas Disease in the Southern Cone of South America," *Millions Saved: Proven Successes in Global Health* (Washington, DC: Center for Global Development, 2004), https://www.cgdev.org/page/case-12-controlling-chagas-disease-southern-cone-south-america.

50 Ibid.
51 Ibid, 6.
52 Jorge Ramírez, et al., "Chile's Role in Global Health Diplomacy."
53 Some relevant selected readings relevant: James Howe, *The Kuna Gathering: Contemporary Village Politics in Panama* (Austin: University of Texas Press, 1986); James Howe, *A People Who Would Not Kneel: The United States and the San Blas Kuna* (Washington, DC: Smithsonian Institute Press, 1998); James Howe, *Chiefs, Scribes & Ethnographers: Kuna Culture from inside and out* (Austin: University of Texas Press, 2009).
54 David Taplin et al., "A Comparative Trial of Three Treatment Schedules for the Eradication of Scabies," *Journal of American Academy of Dermatology* 9 (1983): 550–554, doi:10.1016/s0190-9622(83)70168-4.
55 Today the spelling Niadup is used interchangeably with the more current spelling, Niadub.
56 David Taplin et al., "Community Control of Scabies: A Model Based on Use of Permethrin Cream," *The Lancet* 337, no. 8748 (1991): 1016–1018, doi:10.1016/0140-6736(91)92669-s.
57 On December 20, 1989, President George W Bush authorized a military invasion of Panama to oust General Manuel Noriega. Noriega, surrendered on January 3, 1990, and thereafter was imprisoned in the United States and France for drug trafficking. Ultimately, he was returned to Panama as a prisoner where he died on May 29, 2017. Among the most heinous of Noriega's crimes was the 1985 torture and beheading of political opponent, Dr. Hugo Spadafora, a former Vice-Minister of Health.
58 Taplin et al., "Community Control of Scabies: A Model Based on Use of Permethrin Cream," 1991.
59 Portions of this case study include information from the short article "Cuba in the Time of Cholera & Dengue: A Paradox in Global Health Diplomacy," by Sherri L. Porcelain, *ICCAS: Focus on Cuba* (online), October 2012.
60 Robert V. Tauxe, Eric D. Mintz, and Robert E. Quick, "Epidemic Cholera in the New World: Translating Field Epidemiology into New Prevention Strategies," *Emerging Infectious Diseases* 1, no. 4 (1995): 141–146, doi:10.3201/eid0104.950408.
61 Sherri L. Porcelain, "Cuba in the Time of Cholera."
62 United Nations World Tourism Organization Report, 2012.
63 Roberto Tapia-Conyer, Miguel Betancourt-Cravioto, and Jorge Méndez-Galván, "Dengue: An Escalating Public Health Problem in Latin America," *Paediatrics and International Child Health* 32, no. S1 (2012): 14–17, http://www.ncbi.nlm.nih.gov/pmc/articles/PMC3381443/, and Maria G. Guzman et al., "Dengue: A Continuing Global Threat," *Nature Reviews Microbiology* 8 (2010): S7–S16.
64 Fredi Alexander, Díaz-Quijano, and Eliseu Alves Walman, "Factors Associated with Dengue Mortality in Latin America and the Caribbean, 1995–2009: An Ecological Study," *The American Journal of Tropical Medicine and Hygiene* 86, no. 2 (2012): 328–340, doi:10.4269/ajtmh.2012.11-0074.
65 Jennifer Schneider and Deborah Droll, "A Timeline for Dengue in the Americas to December 31, 2000, and Noted First Occurrences," *Pan American Health Organization* (June 2001), https://www.paho.org/hq/dmdocuments/2010/Atimelinefordengue.pdf.
66 Maria G. Guzmán, "Thirty Years after the Cuban Hemorrhagic Dengue Epidemic of 1981," *Revista Cubana de Medicina Tropical* 64, no. 1 (2012). Reprinted in *MEDICC Review* 14, no. 2 (2012), 46–51.
67 Adriana Troyo, et al., "Dengue in Costa Rica: The Gap in Local Scientific Research," *Revista Panamericana de Salud Pública/Pan American Journal of Public Health* 20, no. 5 (2006), doi:10.1590/s1020-49892006001000012.

68 Juan O. Tamayo, "More Cases of Dengue Fever Reported in Eastern Cuba," *The Miami Herald*, August 20, 2012, http://www.miamiherald.com/2012/08/20/2960476/more-dengue-fever-reported-in.html.

69 "Editorial: Dengue in the Americas–Time to Talk," *The Lancet* 250, no. 9076 (1997): 455.

70 Human Rights Watch telephone interview with Dr. Caridad del Carmen Piñon Rodríguez (Dr. Mendoza Rivero's Wife), Santiago de Cuba, June 25, 1998, https://www.hrw.org/reports/1999/cuba/Cuba996-04.htm#P1086_205576.

71 See Dr. Dessy Mendoza Rivero's, *Dengue: La Epidemia Secreta de Fidel Castro* (Washington, DC: Center for a Free Cuba, 2001) for a more detailed account.

72 Pan American Health Organization, "Chikungunya Countries/Territories with Autochthonous Transmission or Imported Cases in the Americas – EW – 2016," accessed February 1, 2016, http://www.paho.org/hq/index.php?option=com_topics&view=rdmore&cid=6917&Itemid=40931&lang=en.

73 Luis Suárez Rosas, "El silencio de epidemiológico y la ética de la Salud Pública cubana," *Revista Cubana de Salud Pública* 39, no. 3 (2013): 524–539.

74 Juan A. B. Belt and Luis Velazquez, *Cuba: Reforming the Power, Telecommunications and Water Sectors During a Transition* (Presentation, Annual Meetings of the Association for the Study of the Cuban Economy (ASCE), Miami, FL, August 2, 2007), http://pdf.usaid.gov/pdf_docs/PNADJ706.pdf.

75 Ibid, citing from CUBAAGUA/Instituto Nacional de Resursos Hídricos, www.hidro.cu.

76 Anonymous personal interviews conducted in Miami, FL, October 10–13, 2012.

77 Portions of this includes information from the short article "U.S. Cuba Cooperation on Ebola: Disgrace or Diplomacy," by Sherri L. Porcelain, *ICCAS: Focus on Cuba* (online), November 13, 2014.

78 Vincanne A. Adams, et al.

79 Dr. Sandy Kuvin founded the Sanford F. Kuvin Center for the Study of Infectious and Tropical Diseases at Hebrew University, Israel, to promote research on infectious diseases and promote health as a bridge to peace. He passed away on February 28, 2015.

Bibliography – Selected Books

Buss Marchiori, Paulo and Tobar, Sebastián. *Health Diplomacy and Global Health*: Latin American Perspectives. Rio de Janeiro: Editora Fiocruz, 2017.

Cockerham, Geoffrey B. *Global Governance and Public Health: Obstacles and Opportunities*. Lanham, MD: Roman & Littlefield, 2018.

Feinsilver, Julie. *Healing the Masses: Cuba Health Politics at Home and Abroad*. Oakland: University of California Press, 1993.

Hershfield, Katherine. *Health Politics, and Revolution in Cuba since 1898*. New York: Routledge, 2009.

Howe, James. *The Kuna Gathering: Contemporary Village Politics in Panama*. Austin: University of Texas Press, 1986.

Howe, James. *A People Who Would Not Kneel: The United States and the San Blas Kuna*. Washington, DC: Smithsonian Institute Press, 1998.

McInnes, Colin and Lee, Kelly. *Global Health & International Relations*. Cambridge: Polity Press, 2012.

Mendoza Rivero, Dessy. *Dengue: La Epidemia Secreta de Fidel Castro*. Washington, DC: Center for a Free Cuba, 2001.

Pierce, John R. and Writer, Jim. *Yellow Jack: How Yellow Fever Ravaged America and Walter Reed Discovered Its Deadly Secrets*. Hoboken, NJ: John Wiley, 2005.

Rosskam, Ellen and Kickbusch, Ilona, eds. *Negotiating and Navigating Global Health: Case Studies in Global Health Diplomacy*. London: World Scientific Publishing Co, 2012.

Spooner, Mary Helen and Ullmann, Steven. *Cuban Health Cate: Utopia Dreams, Fragile Future*. Lanham, MD: Rowman & Littlefield Publishing Group, 2014.

6
HEALTH SECURITY

The principles of peace, security, and cooperation are the foundation of the World Health Organization (WHO) constitution and inherent to a post-World War II international health strategy. The WHO constitution was founded upon the assumption that "[T]he health of all peoples is fundamental to the attainment of peace and security and is dependent upon the fullest co-operation of individuals and states."[1] The WHO became a specialized agency of the United Nations (UN) in 1948 as "a powerful instrument forged by peace," to assist the war-torn countries.[2] By pairing health issues with peace and security, the signatories of the WHO constitution understood that disease coupled with poverty and other social ills could threaten societies and destabilize governments.[3] Unambiguously, the origin of the first worldwide public health organization was ideologically based on peace, security, and cooperation beyond one nation and only health actors.

Branding a specific public health issue as a social justice, human rights, humanitarian, development, or security concern is not a modern-day controversy. Such perspectives draw upon different actors and different strategies that are influenced by the social, cultural, economic, political, environmental, and technological determinants. Still, 72 years after the founding of the global health system, people appear flummoxed that a multifaceted public health issue could become politicized. This is true for communicable or noncommunicable diseases, intentional or unintentional injuries, or mental health concerns. In the early 1990s, our field team was working on a cholera educational program for indigenous populations in Latin America, and no one ever asked if our intent was to protect social justice or human rights, promote humanitarianism, or adopt a health security strategy. Nevertheless, there is a growing security-based approach, a politicization against the backdrop of increasing

DOI: 10.4324/9781003007401-7

populism, nationalism, fear, and misinformation and purposeful disinformation influencing behaviors across state and non-state actors in the Americas.
The politicization of health issues may be further compromised by a polariza-
tion of ideologies, and where security provides a path to achieve greater political will from local to global levels.

Prioritizing one health or health-related issue over another may have been
recognized more than 100 years ago. It is these beliefs and moral differences
from which the intersection between the security of the state and the security
of people has led us to what we know today as health security. The rise of
health security coincided with a paradigm shift away from traditional security
studies where the state is the object of security and where people within communities are threatened by things such as outbreaks of infectious diseases,[4] and
towards a human security perspective where public health is well situated.

This chapter will explore the securitization of public health using examples
from Latin America and the Caribbean. There are many facets of health security; however, I selected the relationship of security with newly emerging and
re-emerging infectious diseases in the Americas. This will also include a brief
discussion on antimicrobial resistance (AMR) as one of the greatest global public health threats today and the role of biosecurity and biosafety associated with
naturally occurring, unintentional or the intentional spread, deadly pathogens.
To begin, it is useful to explore the assent toward the study of health security.

The WHO/Pan American Health Organization (PAHO) definition of
health, as the state of complete physical, mental, and social well-being and
not merely the absence of disease or infirmity, has been widely accepted since
the 1950s within the medical and public health fields. More recently, broad-
ening the study of health within world affairs provides a wider range of views
from humanitarian and human rights, social justice and reducing health disparities, global public good, economic development coupled with proliferation
of technology, disease prevention, control and research, business interests from
pharmaceutical companies and insurance markets, foreign policy issues, health
diplomacy, and international agreements for security.[5]

Coupling the term health with security is not new, especially as it relates
to the spread of highly infectious diseases. More recently, however, a health
security analysis is used for such things as global obesity, cancer, unintentional,
and intentional injuries where collective violence against ethnic, religious, and
gender-based populations also requires greater attention. Evidence-based research to protect at-risk populations and defend against unintended outcomes
of discrimination or marginalization from stringent security or security-related
policies has important implications. It is the biosecurity of re-emerging and
newly emerging diseases, AMR, and biosafety that seem to generate greatest health security priorities. Nevertheless, health security requires more
evidence-based research to advance the analytical and practical approaches to
prevent, control, and respond to infectious diseases within and across borders,[6]

which may further contribute to the insecurity of populations. For example, in Chapter 4, disasters and climate crisis, the topic of food insecurity in the Dry Corridor of the Northern Triangle of Central America, demonstrate why a wider lens is necessary to understand the economic, political, environmental, and technological determinants that contribute to insecurity and lead to increased hunger, malnutrition, and worse, death.

Health security will benefit from greater clarification in how terms are used and applied within the study of global and regional affairs. This is necessary since academia continues to promote cross-discipline training, such as history of medicine or public health, with anthropology, geography, or international affairs, as well as the study of medical anthropology, medical geography, or global health policy and international and regional affairs. The cross-discipline research presents new approaches, as well as new academic challenges. Consequently, it is instructive to elucidate how terms can be applied with new pedagogical arguments and policy directions endorsing global health security. As we have seen in previous chapters, language matters and yet we struggle to operationalize terms. Stakeholders may have the same desired goal to protect and promote human welfare; yet, the objectives and strategies to achieve this may not be as clear. "Human security is like 'sustainable development' – everyone is for it, but few people have a clear idea of what it means."[7]

Clarity in Terms

From Human to Health Security

The 1994 United Nations Development Program's (UNDP) Human Development Report (HDR) set in motion the call to redefine traditional security with greater attention to human security. Accepting that "everyone has the right to life, liberty and security of person," the UN Declaration of Human Right, Article 3, proposed two main components of human security: "first, safety from sudden chronic threat as hunger, disease, and repression. And second, it means protection from such sudden and hurtful disruptions in the patterns of daily life... " at the family, employment, or community level.[8] The HDR was the first to provide a comprehensive discussion on human security as the essential components of economic, food, health, environmental, personal, community, and political security. This was a concerted effort to shift focus from nation-state security to the security of people and communities with people centered, safety and survival, opportunity, dignity, autonomy, and human rights as core elements, according to the Joint United Nations Programme on HIV/AIDS (UNAIDS).[9]

The human security paradigm[10,11] uses new methodologies to prevent, mitigate, and respond to security challenges. The objective of human security is "to safeguard the vital core of human lives from critical pervasive threats, in a way that is consistent with long term human fulfillment,"[12] along with the acceptance that responding to disease, disaster, genocide, war, terrorism, and economic insecurity are all fundamental to attaining human security.

To achieve this, human security proposed more robust partnerships across governmental, nongovernmental, business, and local to global citizen cooperation. Protecting "the vital core of all human lives in ways that enhance human freedoms and human fulfillment"[13] respects broader approaches. This has been operationalized through the Millennium Development Goals (MDGs) and even more so through Sustainable Development Goals (SDGs), both discussed thoroughly in Chapter 2, showing the shift toward development, peace, human rights, and security that required growing partnerships. Nevertheless, researchers, policymakers, and practitioners struggle to strike the right balance and effectively respond to real-world problems that threaten the livelihoods of peoples. Consequently, the shift to recognize public health as a security issue rather than one based on human rights or human development fell in line with a growing acceptance of human security approaches during the past few decades.

More rapid and further spread of communicable and noncommunicable diseases was discussed in Chapter 3 "Globalization and Public Health". In this chapter, we see how globalization studies can include security perspectives. Sakiko Fukuda-Parr suggests how globalization and human security studies can offer greater insights into insecurities such as global crime, human trafficking, instability of financial markets, job security, spread of diseases, internal conflicts, as well as economic, political, and technological forces of information and communications.[14] The concept of health security became more relevant with growing global interdependence and the increasing concern that an outbreak in one region could impact other parts of the world, especially in areas poorly prepared to respond. By the late 20th century, the necessity to monitor viral spreads became more and more controversial linking science with policy, as Stephen Morse called for better ways to define international rules of spreading viral traffic.[15]

William Aldis reviewed 300 publications, conducted interviews, and identified policies related to the terms health and security. Aldis found the consistent variable was the actors involved.[16] As mentioned at the start of this chapter, the multilateral system of the WHO, a specialized agency of the UN, was always grounded in health and security of peoples as fundamental to their mission. The UNDP first promoted human security in the 1990s, proposing more sustainable development could be achieved if health is accepted as a security matter. This is especially noteworthy in the case of HIV/AIDS, where the UNDP, UNAIDS, WHO, and other key actors involved in HIV/AIDS waivered from humanitarianism, human rights, and development, with a shift toward health security.

Framing Health Security

The most predominant health security concerns are associated with this transborder spread of microbes. Brown and Chalk provide five considerations:

(1) disease threatens human life such that more people die from disease than from war or violence; (2) disease left unchecked threatens the confidence in the state's role; (3) disease threatens the economic system from which human and state security depends; (4) disease can create regional instability such as the case of HIV/AIDS in the sub-Sahara region; and (5) disease, through the threats of bioterrorism or biowarfare, can play a very important strategic role in state policy.[17]

At the World Health Assembly meeting in 2001, an epidemiologic alert system for infectious diseases was created with the intent to improve health security. It was six years later, on World Health Day, April 7, 2007, for the first time the WHO/PAHO selected a theme to connect health with security: *A Safer Future: Global Health Security in the 21st Century*. The controversy on using the term health security arose later that year during an Intergovernmental Meeting (2007) on the Pandemic Influenza Virus, where the debate centered on the security for whom. Defining global health security depended upon agreeing to specific wording that could foster greater cooperation across countries and regions. For example, Portugal wanted a global health security term that would replace pre-existing laws. This was opposed by Brazil, Thailand, Indonesia, and India who refused the inclusion of such language on global health security. The controversy continued, as previously discussed in Chapter 5 on public health diplomacy and the public health security challenge, with Indonesia's declaration to maintain viral sovereignty over their influenza strains.

Public health continues to grow as an important topic in world affairs; therefore, examining the dominant paradigms of international relations theory, such as realism, liberalism, and constructivism, could be useful to understanding how public health is or is not prioritized. Youde suggests that it is not necessary to create a new paradigm for health security; rather use the existing international relations theories,[18] which was further analyzed in the work of McInnes and Lee.[19] In international relations theory, realism and neorealism are based upon traditional security studies where the state is the only key actor and military power is used to protect the state. Liberalism and neoliberalism go beyond the state to include other non-state actors and the important role of economic integration. It appears that constructivism, where the analysis focuses on the changing perceptions depending upon how the issue is framed, may best explain the shift to global public health security. Perceptions about the threat of a public health issue like Ebola, SARS, or Zika virus alter the way we respond to events within the international system and reveal how public health has become increasingly important to foreign policy matters in contemporary times.[20]

Perspectives about managing old and new public health challenges in world affairs have evolved overtime and are fundamental to how policymakers decide to frame an issue. As discussed in Chapter 5 "Health Diplomacy", there is a preponderance of evidence to support why some level of transborder cooperation is necessary. Using science-based policies for health security has become a key element of global health governance. Labonté and Gagnon present six policy frames used for global health and foreign affairs from security, development, global public goods, trade, human rights, and ethical and moral reasoning. In their review of key documents, they found that security and development were the dominant frames.[21] Many may question that securitizing public health issues over framing them as a human right, health equity, development, or humanitarian concerns will neglect a global moral and ethical reasoning to protect the health, safety, and security of populations. This is likely based on the history of security studies where the level of analysis was on protecting the state and not the community or individual.

Traditional security studies have focused on the power of the military as a key actor within and across nations. However, joint military operations are also associated with peace keeping, disaster response, and relief operations. Noteworthy is that militaries leave their countries and are deployed in often harsh conditions in which the troops' safety and health could be at risk. During military operations to an emergency event, the potential contact with highly contagious disease poses an increased threat to the troops as well as to the communities where they return. Therefore, military microbe surveillance and collaboration became an important component of health security. Militaries have assisted with early warning systems through their medical research units and institutes of medical sciences. Public health surveillance through the WHO/PAHO Collaborating Centers and ministries of health in countries may also have the benefit of scientific expertise such as through department of defense international laboratories. For example, since 1983 the Peruvian Navy hosts the U.S. Naval Medical Research Center Detachment (NMRCD) where a strong relationship exists across militaries and with the Ministry of Health.[22] Military-to-military and military-to-civilian partnerships have become more relevant as health security is prioritized.

Case Study 6.1

History of the Field Epidemiology Survey Team (FEST): From Vietnam to Latin America

The history of the Field Epidemiology Survey Team (FEST) is presented to contextualize field research and how it offers unique challenges, unexpected partnerships, and exceptional opportunities to understand and disentangle complex matters where security may play a central role. The FEST may have started on the front lines during the Vietnam War, but it transitioned into a civilian research and community-based public health field work in Latin America.

On September 26, 1966, the FEST unit was created as part of the United States army medical research team in Saigon, composed of Special Forces and technical specialists. Team members were trained at Fort Bragg, North Carolina, and Walter Reed Army Institute of Research (WRAIR), Washington, D.C., with a specific focus on infectious diseases such as malaria, plague, typhus, leptospirosis, schistosomiasis, filariasis, and skin infections. Field epidemiology, historically referred to as "shoe leather" epidemiology, is traced to John Snow's pivotal work in 1850 where he identified the source of cholera epidemic in London. Epidemiology developed to become the science of public health that analyzes the distribution and spread of diseases, injuries, and deaths. The original WRAIR/FEST unit stands out for two reasons. First, it profiles an exemplary military-civilian research collaboration to improve field research methods that would reduce the debilitating infectious diseases of military personnel. Second, it establishes the role field epidemiology can play in the early identification and response to public health threats from military to civilian populations. This field research model, while developed for military units in Vietnam, was later adapted for field research teams in Latin America.

According to Dr. Al Allen, the WRAIR/FEST concept was the brainchild of U.S. Army Major, Colonel Llewellyn J. (Lew) Legters, a preventive medicine officer of the U.S. John F. Kennedy Center for Special Warfare at Fort Bragg, North Carolina. In the mid-1960s, Major Legters, a Green Beret of Special Forces, reasoned that the U.S. military needed better field research strategies to identify diseases that might afflict personnel on military operations in Vietnam across the diverse terrain of the Mekong Delta.[23] Major Legters proposed a unique plan to train Special Forces to collect blood, skin, and vector samples from forward combat areas, rather than have scientists wait for samples to arrive at their laboratory clinics and hospitals. This exemplifies "shoe leather" epidemiology and the preventive public health practice. This work has been documented in medical journals and in an official military medical history book contributing greatly to our knowledge of diseases of military importance.[24]

Col. Legters brought WRAIR/FEST to life, but he did not work alone. Then Captain, retired Colonel Alfred M. Allen, conducted research on skin-related health issues with combat forces, supporting troops, and civilian populations in the Mekong Delta. Mobile field laboratories, with special culture media, were able to isolate microbes that previously went undetected by traditional methods. In less than six months new approaches for the prevention and treatment of health risks in the field among military population were realized.[25] The most frequent causes of skin-related infections and disabilities where troops in Vietnam often spent three or more days in wet terrain. These field studies contributed to the future research in other ecological niches with mobile military troops around the globe, leading to important field research conducted in the Western Hemisphere.

FEST Transition from Military to Academia

Col. Allen, along with civilian scientists from the University of Miami field teams, trained in the Florida Everglades National Park, a wet terrain that could simulate conditions in the Mekong Delta. This training took place under the supervision of the University of Miami Medical School's, Dr. Harvey Blank, a dermatologist along with Professor David Taplin, a field research scientist who studied infections and infestations of the skin. The Vietnam War research found that 50% of the field forces were affected with skin diseases. This created a unique opportunity to conduct valuable research of military and civilian significance. An obstacle, as evidenced today, is maintaining an adequate supply chain of necessary materials. This was exacerbated by "growing military bureaucracy, administrative 'red tape,' and a relatively slow supply system within Vietnam, forced FEST to find unique and sometimes bizarre ways of circumventing the system."[26] However, I can say confidently that the "bizarre ways" were no match for the creative genius of Taplin in the field (Figure 6.1).

In 1968, Taplin traveled with the military forces to help create a field base laboratory in the Mekong Delta, followed by the teams who

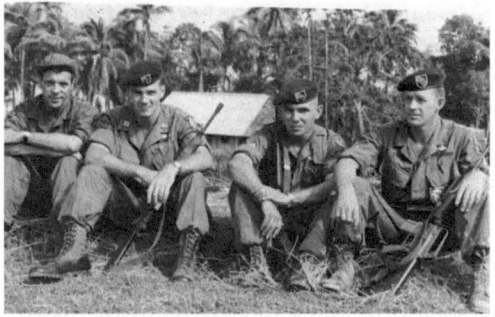

FIGURE 6.1 The Original Military-Civilian Field Epidemiology Survey Team (FEST) Members from L to R David Taplin, Captain Alfred M. Allen, Sergeant First Class Robert E. Weaver, Staff Sergeant Ray A. Drewry, South Vietnam (1968). Photo Credits: FEST archives, donated to S. Porcelain, 2010.

conducted studies in Vietnam, Thailand, Uganda, Panama, Venezuela, and Colombia.[27] However, in 1975 the military component of the FEST was disbanded; Taplin then created the University of Miami's FEST. And I was offered extraordinary opportunities, lasting decades, inspiring me to see things differently than I could have ever imagined allowing me to understand the nexus of health and security.

Taplin championed the scientific research for practical field application and brought an adapted FEST model to the University of Miami Miller School of Medicine, Departments of Dermatology and Epidemiology and Public Health with a focus on Latin America and the Caribbean. A mobile and self-sufficient field team was formed. The FEST, in collaboration with national and international military units, as well as community and indigenous populations to reduce risks of infections and infestations conducting studies, targeted community health programs, disaster and emergency response, and innovative public health educational strategies. These wide-ranging partnerships expanded across the ministries of health in host countries, local community members, health providers, other researchers, scholars, practitioners, nongovernmental and community-based organizations, and industry. These partnerships created unique opportunities to conduct novel research and support public health policy recommendations. Cultivating science for evidence-based policy became part of the FEST overall goal. However, through it all, we tried not to lose sight that the complexities of this field research extended well beyond the medical and public health fields. This is the space I felt most comfortable, respecting the broader context of population health, to include the political, economic, social, cultural, environmental, ecological, and technological determinants as well as ethical and moral reasoning that are essential to meeting such challenges today. I found an appropriate fit, as a nonmedical person asking questions when there were clearly no easy answers, and often well beyond narrow limits of a specific health issue.

Conclusion

The FEST conducted research and community-based programs, with an emphasis on Central and South America. A permanent field research station was established in Panama in the early 1980s. Ultimately, the tropical dermatology focus transitioned into community-based health, disasters, and community development partnerships in the Latin America and Caribbean region. The FEST evolved over the years to become part of a global public health program that slowly came to an end in 2008.

Case Study 6.2

Reflections of Public Health Security – Barrancabermeja, Colombia

As my first introduction to Colombia took place in the capital city of Bogotá in the late 1970s, my second was as a graduate student studying tropical infectious diseases of the skin in a more remote region of the country and a new member of the Field Epidemiology Survey Team (FEST). The crossroads of health and security in the early through mid-1980s were palpable from the start.

Our research was in collaboration with mobilizing Colombian military troops stationed in an oppressively hot and humid region situated on the Magdalena River outside the city of Barrancabermeja. The city is best known for its oil fields, and at that time as a terrorist refuge. The locals introduced their city to me in its shortened version, *Barranca*, known for its three P's in Spanish: *Petrol, Prostitución, y Plata*. (Petroleum, Prostitution, and Money). Others referred to *Barranca* as the armpit of Colombia. I soon realized *Barranca* would be a complex environment.

Field Research

I saw soldiers as young as 17 years of age, many from poverty-stricken communities, forced to combat more than their human foe. Their battle against the pesky mosquitoes that transmitted malaria and dengue fever, as well as the creeping crusted and debilitating fungal infections of the body, groin, and feet, left many of these young men incapacitated. They were unable to wear compulsory military uniforms or combat boots due to excruciatingly inflamed skin. This was not the ordinary athlete's foot, a type of fungal infection we are most familiar with, and where such itching and burning are easily treated with a spray or a cream to kill the fungus. We were studying aggressive fungal infections that spread throughout the body, groin, and feet and were occurring in nature not in gyms or dormitory bathrooms, which are associated with the outbreaks in the United States. In partnership with the Colombian military, we conducted field-based clinical trials on new topical creams and systemic treatments developed by Janssen Pharmaceutical, called Ketoconazole, a next-generation antifungal agent to treat the rapidly spreading fungal infections. This translation of field-based research for appropriate military policies was modeled after the original field unit in Vietnam for United States troops.[28] This brought about significant changes in the types of clothing, boots, and behaviors of military troops.

I was fortunate to work under the direction of David Taplin, University of Miami Professor, Dermatology and Cutaneous Surgery and Epidemiology and Public Health, who developed a specialization in field research as a tropical mycology scientist.[29] I cannot minimize his scientific ingenuity and the immense impact he had on countless researchers, practitioners, and students across many fields of study. He introduced me to the study of field epidemiology, infectious disease research, and how scientific evidence coupled with personal interactions can be used to encourage policymakers to make changes. I learned that skin problems, which may not be the highest priority in global public health, provide good results in a short time. It inspires the heartfelt gratitude and pleasure from populations suffering from intense itching, scratching, and pain disrupting one's ability to work, sleep, or study. This introduction to field epidemiology research was clearly a valuable educational lesson, which extends beyond the scientific study of disease and response to more broadly embrace the politics, social and cultural behaviors, economics, ecological, and environment factors. These are the important determinants to understand poor population health outcomes.

I also learned that skin-related problems, from infections or infestations in tropical and semi-tropical regions, were the cause of great disability. It required improved access to public health infrastructure, education, and early prevention strategies. Second, early intervention could dramatically improve the problem within days, thereby generating good will within a population. This sets the stage for more engaged participation of people to be involved in their own health outcomes. Third, the skin can be photographed to depict changes taking place, allowing individuals to both feel better and observe the dramatic changes. Seeing is believing. Fourth, it promotes an eagerness to take on more public health actions. Fifth, it conveys empathy, which I have come to learn is an essential component of public health life. Lastly, I experienced the benefit of using a camera in public health. It is a valuable education and training tool, as long as it is ethically and culturally tailored to respect all individuals equally. This is where I found great interest, and the most valuable lessons I learned, in taking the time to appreciate the different perspectives that influence how people interact within their community.

A Unique Field Experience, as Most Are

One of the most memorable events, during these field studies from 1980 to 1984, occurred in 1982, while Taplin was away delivering a keynote lecture in his home country, England. Our mobile FEST field team was working with a Battalion in Norte de Santander in the city of Barrancab-ermeja, Colombia in a region of the country that was quickly emerging as a hot spot for violence. Our field research station was located in a house, provided through *Ecopetrol*, Colombia's largest state-owned petroleum company, and situated next to the military barracks. An early knock at our door presented an unusual request from the *Coronel de batallón* (Battalion Colonel). His troops were mobilized atop of a hill and had fallen prey to debilitating spreading fungal infections that required immediate care. If we agreed to go, they warned us that the trip would be difficult, and possibly dangerous.

Did I have any idea of what they proposed as dangerous? We had a very short window of time to prepare. We were armed with field kits of alcohol, scalpels to collect skin scales, glass slides to view the scales under a microscope upon return, potassium hydroxide, antifungal and topical steroid creams along with some essential field supplies of insect repellent, potable water, and meals ready to eat (MREs). A military medic traveled with us so he could assess and treat the men. We suggested the younger field team member to stay behind; however, Sarah Rowsey, the adventurous and inquisitive daughter of Taplin, was eager to participate. It is no surprise she later changed her career path to become a paramedic and first responder.

I soon realized that we would be escorted to a remote location by armed young men toting M19s and other large automatic weapons. Their job was to protect us. After a long, bumpy, and arduous journey we arrived and confronted the worst cases of tropical fungal infections ever imagined. They were in excruciating pain from their raw red scaling skin from head to toe. Consequently, they were unable to actively engage in military maneuvers from this remote staging base of operations. The field team took samples of their skin scales so we could determine the type of fungi, provided the health education on how to apply the antifungal topical treatment along with personal hygiene tips under austere living conditions.

We were already teamed up with the Colombian military on a double-blind clinical trial and had many tubes of open label antifungal creams for serious cases that were not enrolled in this study. We were evaluating how the new treatment compared with the older existing one, and to make sure it was safe and effective. These severe cases fit the protocol. At first, I perceived this as a humanitarian response, albeit an intriguing escapade to the clandestine field military base that became legendary among the soldiers and our team. Clearly, this research opportunity would likely not exist today with health, safety, and security protocols rightfully in place. Upon Taplin's return, and only in his inimitable style, he showed his pleasure with our rapid response. He was quite disappointed that we did not photograph such severe cases. It was unfortunate that smartphones technology did not exist in 1982 and the option of hauling our expensive equipment was not feasible. But he was right. I've learned that a picture, through the lens that one selects, leaves a lasting impression that words cannot fully capture. We did receive word that within days the topical treatments worked, and the young men were back in service.

Conclusion

While I didn't realize it then, this would become my first introduction to the crossroads of health and security. I learned that early identification, rapid surveillance, access to simple and low costs treatments, health education for military units, and small-scale policy changes, such as the issue of sandals and cotton clothing during their downtime, could prevent the debilitating fungal and secondary skin infections. I also learned that social, cultural, political, economic, ecological, and environmental factors were all relevant to understanding the nexus of health and security.

Almost four decades later, the face of public health security endures, threatening populations across the globe with newly emerging and re-emerging infectious diseases. The relationship of health and security, while not new, shows the significance of public -private partnerships across military and civilian collaborations. Since I've had the opportunity to work with military and paramilitary groups, urban and remote communities, rich and poor, I have a much deeper appreciation of the value of partnerships that safeguard the health and security of peoples.

History

As discussed in earlier chapters, the demand to control the spread of diseases from East to West and South to the North required a cooperative response to safeguard the health of nation-states. It has also been argued throughout history that the early motivation for states to cooperate was deeply rooted in protecting maritime states and their economic interests. The motivations to control plague and cholera spreading along trade routes have been questioned. Were actions and policies driven by priorities to protect people or economies, and which people and which economies? The 14th-century Black Death, also known as the bubonic plague, transmitted by fleas living off rats in ships and infecting their human hosts, represents the first-time maritime quarantine practices were implemented in Europe. From plague during the Middle Ages quarantine in Venice, Italy, to the highly infectious measles and smallpox spread from Europe to the New World, efforts to reduce diseases and deaths also triggered questions whether such motivations were to safeguard economic security of the state or security of people?

Are these questions different today? Asking if controlling Zika virus in the Americas was based upon protecting vulnerable at-risk populations within regions such as northern Brazil, or was it more closely associated with the perceived security of economies and livelihoods by other states in the region? States cannot do it alone, and global public health security depends on international cooperation and the willingness of all countries to take steps to tackle new and emerging threats.[30]

Throughout history, microbes have destabilized populations. Historian William McNeill in *Plagues and Peoples*[31] explored how diseases destroyed China, India, and the Mediterranean to Roman Empire to the European conquest of indigenous empires of the Aztec and Incas arrival to Mexico and Peru in the 15th and 16th centuries. His political and ecological analysis provided important insights into how diseases traveled along with people and shaped history, as later in Jared Diamond's *Guns, Germs, and Steel*, where his historical analysis of human evolutions highlights the environment and geography impacts on humanity.[32] McNeill's work explores the significance of ecological factors where infectious diseases became an important determinant in human history.[33] For example, the human-induced impact of desertification is linked to the collapse of the Mayan communities in 800–1000 CE where the stress of social and environmental pressures led to the destructions of populations.[34] McNeill discussed parasites and their relationship to governments from the micro to macro levels. In his human ecology analysis, microparasites are the pathogens and macroparasites are how governments respond to such parasites, demonstrating the important intersection of science and policy for health security.

David Fidler coined the term germ governance to describe how societies have responded to microbial challenges within and beyond their porous national borders, considering newly identified diseases and the return of older diseases. Fidler uses an historical perspective to show how germ governance has transformed from a horizontal to a more vertical form of governance.[35] His analysis suggests that the horizontal forms of government existed from the mid-19th century until the end of World War II when infectious diseases were considered external threats to a nation and could be mitigated by encouraging and maintaining international cooperation in trade and travel. During the post-World War II era a more vertical form of governance focused on the spread of disease internally rather than a focus of concern on the external threats. This was based upon human rights approaches that emphasized strengthening a nations' public health infrastructure and providing better primary health care. By the 1990s, more participation from non-state actors became important to the process of global health governance. The 1990s brought worldwide attention to public health in world affairs with a focus on HIV/AIDS along with tuberculosis and malaria. The WHO's IHR declined in importance as the World Trade Organization (WTO), World Bank (WB), and International Monetary Fund (IMF) increased their role in global health matters, and regionally with the PAHO and the Inter-American Development Bank (IDB). HIV/AIDS and human rights approaches gained momentum with Brazil's leadership in securing compulsory licensing for lifesaving HIV/AIDS drugs through the WTO Trade-Related Intellectual Property Rights (TRIPS), as discussed previously in Chapter 3.

Rise of Health Security

The end of the Cold War set forth new forms of conflict that were no longer among states but occurring within states where violence and displacement emerged as key threats to the health, safety, and security of peoples. This includes civil conflicts and increasingly displaced populations where the role of bipolar powers to maintain the balance no longer existed. This presented the changing perceptions of security with shifting geopolitical factors corresponding to the new threats within and across regional borders. Health security became more important to regional and international affairs with a greater understanding that the "ordinary dynamics of international relations and the specific dynamics produced by the challenged posed by pathogenic microbes."[36] Deadly pathogens became reframed as existential threats that required international political responses to protect populations and the world economy.[37] This brought many new actors, new underlying issues, and a health security perspective to the larger issues in world affairs. The international collaborators' effort to prevent and reduce the spread of diseases, such as HIV/AIDS, malaria, tuberculosis to name a few, may have been motivated by passionate pleas for global engagement based upon humanitarian and ethical principles, or the eager efforts to promote a country's self-interest.

Global Health Security Actions

The Global Health Security Initiative began as an informal group with the European Union, France, Germany, Italy, Japan, Mexico, United Kingdom, and United States meeting in Ottawa, Canada in November 2001 to "strengthen health preparedness and response globally to threats of biological, chemical, radio nuclear terrorism (CBRN) and pandemic influenza."[38] This initiative was based upon building a country's capacity to deter the spread of diseases through the advances in laboratory and epidemiologic surveillance.[39]

The launch of the Global Health Security Agenda (GHSA) in February 2014 set forth an expanded collaborative effort for countries to meet challenges associated with development, globalization and food supply, travel, microbial resistance, and the spread of microbes. The GHSA focused on building a nation's capacity to prevent, detect, and respond as a best practice for health security whether the pathogen threat is naturally occurring, intentional, or caused by human error such as breaches in laboratory research. This means funding scientific training, building better laboratories, improving epidemiologic surveillance with the necessary local to national partnerships. From the start, participating countries in this hemisphere included Argentina, Canada, Mexico, and the United States.

> As of September 2018, 65 participating countries representing nearly 6 billion people, along with 9 international and regional multilateral organizations and institutions, and non-governmental sector partners – including over 100 private companies, non-governmental organizations, and academic institutions are part of GHSA.[40]

The new global health security vision focused on a safe and secure world with greater attention to the early identification of zoonotic (animal to human) infectious disease threats. In 2017, participating member states presented a five-year strategy, through the Kampala Declaration until 2024. At the GHSA Meeting hosted by Thailand on November 20, 2020, global health security gaps were identified with a clear urgency to respond to the coronavirus pandemic. To meet these needs, the GHSA 2024 would require more sectors and more stakeholders to collaborate and cooperate to sustain common goals for global health security.[41]

The creation of the Global Health Security Index (GHSI) is a new joint effort with the Nuclear Threat Initiative (NTI), Johns Hopkins University (JHU) Center for Health Security, and Economist Intelligence Unit (EIU). The GHS Index is the first comprehensive approach to measure changes in national health security across 195 nations with the intended purpose of improving global capacity to respond to an epidemic or pandemics, which could be due to naturally occurring, intentional, unintentional actions such as gaps in laboratory safety. Each organization brings different points of reference to study security threats.[42]

> Overall, the GHS Index finds severe weaknesses in country abilities to prevent, detect, and respond to health emergencies; severe gaps in health systems; vulnerabilities to political, socioeconomic, and environmental risks that can confound outbreak preparedness and response; and a lack of adherence to international norms.[43]

In 2019, in a global health security study of 195 countries, no country was found to be fully prepared, with an overall scale of 40.2 out of 100 and an average of

51.9 in high-income countries. Countries were rated on their readiness to prevent, detect, respond, health norms, and risk. According to the Global Health Security Initiative (GHSI), the top ten countries prepared in Latin America were Brazil ranked the highest at 59.7, followed by Argentina (58.6), Chile (58.3), Mexico (57.6), Ecuador (50.1), Peru (49.2), Costa Rica (45.1), Colombia and El Salvador both (44.2), and Panama (43.7).[44] The United States ranked first out of 195 countries scoring 89.3 for biosecurity and 100 for biosafety, with an overall average of 83.5 compared to the lowest in the world, Equatorial Guinea's 195/195 index score 16.2.[45] Such indicators used for assessing readiness will need further scrutiny as we reflect upon the disastrous COVID-19 response from the highest ranked country, the United States.

Newly Emerging and Re-Emerging Diseases

A newly emerging infectious disease is one that has never been identified before, while a re-emerging disease has existed in a specific region before it was eliminated — and now reappears in new areas where at times the microbes are resistant to the drugs previously used. As presented earlier in the book, more than 70% of the newly emerging diseases are zoonotic. This means they originate in animals and jump species when they infect humans, followed by human-to-human transmission. The re-emergence in the Americas of old disease threats such as cholera and yellow fever, dengue, malaria, and tuberculosis, the threats of drug resistance to malaria or co-infections of HIV/AIDS, and the re-emergence of tuberculosis face drug resistance and multidrug resistance in the region.[46] Securitizing these public health problems intersects with economies, environment, trade, tourism, international workers, military forces deployed overseas, and a political justification to respond. The end of the 20th century further pushed health toward security as seen with HIV/AIDS.

Securitization of HIV/AIDS

HIV/AIDS set forth an arduous securitization approach, moving it from low to high politics on the global agenda. In his essay, *The Politics of Health in the Eighteenth Century*, Michel Foucault described how European arguments about the role of biopolitics and biopower are helpful to understand the securitization of HIV/AIDS in more recent times. A biopolitical approach introduces how the biological characteristics of a specific population become a security issue; therefore, it justifies using rigorous research to collect surveillance and monitoring data on a specific population for the purpose of reducing the threat. Foucault portrayed biopolitics in the 18th century, expanding its reach into politics across issues of war and peace to include human health, well-being, and extending life expectancy.[47] Biopower is applied to how governments would then use strategies to protect population health. However, the inevitable unintended consequences have been seen when bad research leads to spurious correlations and poor decisions. The HIV/AIDS epidemic, as seen earlier in history in the case of syphilis, exposed how blaming, shaming, and stigmatizing populations further exacerbated health inequities and its relevancy to the social determinants of health. In the early 1980s HIV/AIDS research in the Northern Hemisphere focused its attention on specific populations identified as the 4-Hs: heroin users, homosexuals, hemophiliacs, and Haitians. Using imperfect research methods, an unfortunate stigmatization of the Haitian people and their economy occurred.

The response to the HIV/AIDS epidemic in resource poor countries began with a humanitarian and human rights approach, then shifted to health and economic development, and expanded to include health security strategies, while maintaining that HIV/AIDS was closely associated with social and health inequalities. The impact on Latin America and the Caribbean was far-reaching. According to the UN AIDS data, the Caribbean became the second most affected region in the world after Africa and the leading cause of death of 15–44 year olds with women 51% of the cases in 2005. Trinidad and Tobago's HIV positive rates were five times higher for girls than boys in the age range of 15–24.[48]

The historic January 10, 2000 United Nations Security Council (UNSC) meeting became the first time a public health issue was ever presented before the council. Resolution 1308 placed HIV/AIDS squarely into the security agenda, and compelled nations to prioritize HIV as a deadly virus that could destabilize sub-Saharan Africa and other regions, creating political and economic upheaval within and across regions. At the same time, with mandatory reporting of AIDS cases in Latin America, the most active surveillance underway was taking place in Costa Rica and Peru. During early 2000s different patterns of disease transmission were seen in Latin America, with men having sex with men (MSM), intravenous drug users, and commercial sex workers at the highest risk; however, it also spread to the wider general population in Honduras and Brazil's southeastern region. According to the World Bank 2000 data, since the late 1980s Latin America had a good capability of responding to HIV/AIDS at the community level by engaging strong partnerships, even though issues of access to health care and stigmatization of high-risk population continue.[49] However, the re-emergence of tuberculosis (TB) and the co-infections associated with HIV/AIDS became an increasing security issue with drug and multidrug resistance to TB.

While there is less research on small states in the Caribbean, a thoughtful analysis by Wendy Grenade examines the securitization of HIV/AIDS and its relationship to tourism, and sustainable development using the case study of Grenada. One view is that securitizing HIV/AIDS through any negative publicity will cause a decline in tourism and lead to significant economic losses. This is important since the Caribbean is one of the most tourist-dependent regions in the world. The second view considers the potential danger tourists may bring to the country, thereby threatening population health security. Ultimately, Grenade concludes that there are both internal and external factors to consider in the intersection of the dependency on tourism, threat of HIVAIDS, and sustainable development.[50] This is important since research shows that countries with economies dependent upon tourism had some of the highest prevalence and incidence rates of HIV/AIDS in the region[51] and where sex tourism is an important factor.

Some argued that HIV/AIDS was too depended on biomedical aspects and not enough on the political, economic, and social structures of societies. Lee and Zwi (1996) and Denis Altman (1999) suggested more rigorous study of the relationship of the global economic and political processes beyond the epidemiology of HIV/AIDS. HIV/AIDS would benefit from the principles of global political economy with inclusion of ethical and practical approaches.[52] There were various prevention and mitigation strategies used around the world, and the most provocative actions may have taken place in Cuba.

HIV was first identified in Cuba in 1985 among military troops returning home from Africa. In 1986, with increasing cases among the civilian gay population, mandatory HIV testing was initiated throughout Cuban society, and anyone identified as HIV positive was placed in a sanitarium where they were guarded by military personnel and not permitted to leave unless they were escorted for short visits to their homes. Patients received "comfortable rooms and good food and medical and personal attention, but their personal liberty was severely restricted."[53] Three years later controls were eased; yet it wasn't until the early 1990s that those infected with HIV were able to move more freely to receive outpatient care.[54] The argument that such actions violated human rights has been juxtaposed to Cuba reporting one of the lowest rates of HIV in the world. No matter where you stand on the issue, the moral and ethical reasoning of protecting an individual over the collective populations well-being continues to direct actions to control and reduce the spread of infectious diseases within different political systems, e.g. Ebola, and COVID-19 today.

One of the greatest global public health achievements in history began with U.S. President George W Bush's 2002 State of the Union address of the President's Emergency Plan for AIDS Relief (PEPFAR) calling for $15 billion to combat HIV/AIDS. Was the new policy motivated by humanitarianism and a moral responsibility, human rights and social equity, concern for economic development, or a security threat? Was it the star power of well-informed international musicians Bono Vox (U2) and fellow Irishman David Geldof who led the fight to make poverty history, that presented the HIV/AIDS message to the U.S. Congress, or was it the economic and political security threat that motivated a response? The social disintegration of societies due to increasing mortality among wage earners, along with the emotional images of dying mothers and children, and further economic and political instability were all identified as different points of view. Securitizing HIV/AIDS created the greatest motivation for action through the UN Security Council. Depending upon which stakeholder you ask, with their different viewpoints, the urgency for new strategies, better access to lifesaving drugs, and new partnerships came to fruition for a robust global security response to HIV/AIDS.

H1N1 Swine Flu

In spring 2009, H1N1 influenza pandemic became a top political priority in the Americas and beyond, with an initial fear that this newly identified viral strain could become as deadly as the 1918 H1N1 flu pandemic. This ignited a public health emergency with more than 18,000 deaths across the global. If there is any doubt that the foundation of the WHO/PAHO was both conceptualized and realized within a framework that promotes health and security, look no further than the declaration and the dialogue on pandemic flu. The good news is the 2009 strain was not as virulent. The bad news was that it was easily transmissible. Infected people may not have felt very sick, so they engaged in normally activities, and the virus spread.

The WHO/PAHO asked countries around the world to increase their surveillance, monitoring, and reporting efforts. On April 25, 2009, the IHR implemented a public health emergency of international concern (PHEIC) for H1N1 influenza. Two days later the U.S. Centers for Disease Control and Prevention (CDC) issued travel warnings to Mexico where increasing and more serious cases of influenza and pneumonia were reported. Even with Mexico's commitment to transparency, the reality of uneven economic development across rural communities remained a barrier for people to have access to public health communication efforts.[55]

Through a pre-existing relationship between Canada, Mexico, and the United States, known as the Security and Prosperity Partnership (SPP) of North America Security Agenda, countries were able to share timely information with the PAHO. The SPP of North America Security Agenda was formalized on March 23, 2005 with leaders of the three countries as a

> common security strategy to further secure North America and ensure the streamlined movement of legitimate travelers and cargo across our shared borders. To this end, Canada, the United States, and Mexico will work together to ensure the highest continent-wide security standards and streamlined risk-based border processes are achieved.[56]

The SPP provided a clear mechanism for communicating and sharing information, countering the criticism that each country's motivation would exist simply to protect individual country's national and economic security. Such a borderless public health issue bared the value of the SPP of North America

Security Agenda. Since SARS was identified in 2003, there have been up-dated requirements for reporting infectious diseases of international concern, improved public health communication networks, and the formation of the Global Health Security Action group in the Americas, with all contributing to a well-integrated H1N1 response.

The 2009 swine flu had a significant impact on public health, development, globalization, diplomacy, and security levels in Mexico. It is estimated that the H1N1 epidemic caused a 70% tourist cancellation with hotel occupancy rates dropping from an expected 55% to 15%, while cruise reservations reported a high cancellation rate generating a loss of approximately 134,000 tourists. Argentina and Cuba suspended flights from Mexico,[57] and international con-ferences, a significant contributor to Mexico's economy, reported an additional 47,000 more visitor cancellations. The Minister of Finance, Agustin Carstens, estimated the country would lose US$ 2.2 billion related to the health crisis before Mexico would return to normal activities upon controlling the spread of this influenza.[58] Prioritizing and promoting public health transparency in the end cost Mexico almost $9 billion dollars.[59]

Zika Virus[60]

Zika virus is another viral disease caused by the same mosquito as yellow fever, dengue, and chikungunya. It was first identified in the Zika Forest, Uganda in 1947 with the first human case documented in 1952. It spread to tropic areas in Africa, Southeast Asia, and Pacific Islands and in 2007 it infected 75% of the population in the Pacific Island of Yap. By 2013 it spread to French Polynesia, Cook Islands, and Easter Island. It wasn't until 2015 that it arrived in Brazil spreading rapidly throughout the Americas.

In May 2015, the PAHO confirmed the first case, but suggested it may have arrived earlier in 2014. Two theories on how it reached the Americas suggest different paths: the *Journal of Science* (2016) presents a 2013–2014 link when the epidemic struck French Polynesia and was introduced into Brazil during a soc-cer match, while the *Journal of Community Health* (2016) suggests a 2014–2015 link when it arrived from the Polynesia Islands during a canoe competition in Rio de Janeiro, Brazil. What is worth recognizing is that both theories are associated with globalization and international sporting events taking place in Brazil.

It wasn't until February 1, 2016 that the WHO declared Zika a PHIEC with local transmission and wider spread to new areas in the Americas. The highest rates were reported in poor communities in the northern Brazil, and more spe-cifically in Recife where microcephaly was identified in newborns; Brazil was already suffering from dengue, dengue hemorrhagic fever, and chikungunya. The arrival of Zika virus made controlling mosquitoes an even higher prior-ity. This was about the same time when the country witnessed an increase in yellow fever cases. All such diseases were found in the same mosquito, spreading from Brazil and continued through the Caribbean. Was the commitment to Zika virus based upon the security threat that it would cause transborder havoc especially among pregnant mothers fearing microcephaly? Once again, it depends upon who you ask from scientists, practitioners, politicians, to citizen groups and poor mothers. What we recognize is through robust surveillance and data sharing, the disproportionate impact infected the poor and the social, societal, and environmental determinants which place populations at higher risk. In December 2018, an international genomic study of travelers uncovered a "hidden" Zika virus outbreak, showing "a whole outbreak that had gone undetected." According to the authors, it "demonstrates that the vast majority of Zika cases during 2017 were the result of an unreported Zika outbreak in Cuba."[61]

Public Health Security Research

Will gathering the data improve evidence-based policies for health security? The answer is yes, and no. Unequivocally, evidence-based research is necessary. But it is insufficient without translating the data into useful information, disseminating them timely, safeguarding communication that respects effective, targeted, sensitive, and culturally appropriate public health actions and sound policies. Experts waving their data, cajoling people to act based upon the evidence, will not necessarily achieve the intended outcome of science-based approaches.

An example of field epidemiologic research for evidence-based decision making that would support health security occurred in real time. It was on May 11, 1996 at 2:15 pm when the ValuJet DC-9 plane crashed in Everglades, Florida 17.4 miles west of the Miami International Airport with 110 people abroad. The Everglades virtually digested the aircraft, and all remains in a remote location, with limited access, no infrastructure, in a wet terrain tropical ecosystem. First responders were needed to collect evidence on the cause of the crash to retrieve the voice recorder, better known as the Blackbox. As part of the University of Miami's FEST working in collaboration with the Miami-Dade Task Force first responders, I was tasked with collecting the water and muck samples at the crash site. From day 1, I collected such samples to identify the potential pathogens that could be a health and safety threat to the first responders (Figure 6.2).

The threat was based upon two known facts. First, there was another Everglades, Florida crash on December 29, 1972 when an Eastern Airlines L-1011 jumbo jet crashed and killed 101 with 75 survivors. The FEST members responded, while I did not join the team until eight years later, I learned there were many survivors who died due to gangrene infections. The spectrum of microorganisms in the surrounding uncontaminated area was similar to what

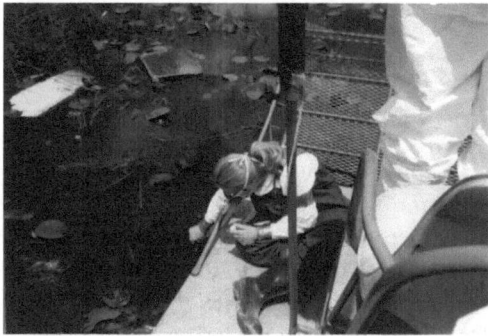

FIGURE 6.2   ValuJet Crash Site: Collecting water and muck samples for antibiotic sensitivities May 1996. Photo from FEST archives, donated to S. Porcelain.

was found in the 1972 L-1011 airplane crash in the Everglades.[62] Second, two weeks prior to the 1996 crash we were teaching an international health field course in the Everglades where one of the student's field project was sampling water and muck 7 miles from this crash site. Therefore, we had recent baseline data of expected pathogens. It was a hot humid time of the year and understanding the ecological niche could provide useful information for other similar ecosystems and potential health and security risks.[63]

This data was useful since we were working in the tropical regions of Latin America. Based upon the scientific evidence collected in and around the crater site from day 1 to 37, the Federal Bureau of Investigation (FBI) cordoned off the area as a public health and security risk to prevent looters from entering by airboats. In and near the crater site we found a very high load of natural Everglades bacteria and those of human origin, including bacteria from intestinal contents. In addition to microbial load, residual jet fuel, lubricants, and hydraulic fuel were a concern for deep penetrated wounds which could become infected due to the irritant nature of the contaminants. The microbiological and antibiotic sensitivities to the gram-negative bacteria associated with humans were identified and a list of antibiotic sensitivities was provided. This research supported evidence-based policies and procedures for health, safety, and security of first responders.

Was the research for health security purposes to protect first responders, potential trespassers, or to use the evidence to protect outsiders from a potential crime scene? In 1996, this crash was determined to be a criminal act of negligence against the maintenance contractor, a cargo company, for failing to train employees, and improper handling and packaging of oxygen canisters. This revolutionized the safety and security of how air cargo is transported today. Further, monitoring the microbiological samples to identify bacterial pathogens and their antibiotic sensitivities was available to ensure any first responder cut by razor-edged sawgrass or other debris had the science to support best treatment and prevent any life-threatening infections that occurred in the

1972 crash. This is even more important today as antimicrobial and antibiotic resistant has become one of the greatest health security threats.

Antibiotic Resistance – Antimicrobial Resistance

AMR may be a silent epidemic, but it is considered one of the greatest public health threats in modern times. Microorganisms that develop AMR are sometimes referred to as "superbugs."[64] Data trends on regional and global AMR may not reflect the danger of AMR. In 2018, the WHO Global Action Plan initiated and prioritized AMR. Dr. Tedros Adhanom Ghebreyesus, Director General of the WHO, shared that 100 countries have a national action plan to respond to this threat, with 50 more countries considering how to proceed. Consequently, in a world with increasing travel, trade, and tourism, AMR presents challenges for all.

It is not the human, animals, or plants that are becoming resistant to the antibiotics; it is the microbe that is more resilient, and the reasons are multi-factorial. Humans, livestock, and terrestrial and aquatic environments confront inappropriate or overuse of antibiotics, requiring further consideration of the disposal, waste, and overall lack of governmental regulations. Governments still have lax policies on antibiotics. Incomplete or inappropriate use of antibiotics may help the bacteria fight back against the medicine that was used to kill the bacteria.[65] The International Federation of Pharmaceutical Manufacturers & Associations (IFPMA) developed a stewardship program with appropriate treatment protocols to promote reporting processes for the misuse of medication. The Food and Agriculture Organization (FAO) of the UN is responsible for both reducing and combating AMR present in agricultural systems. The FAO is currently working on a new resolution, the FAO Action Plan on AMR, which will improve the awareness on AMR through food and agricultural points of view and strengthen governance related to the issue. AMR has become a growing concern in lower-income countries with an increasing demand of meat products and the availability of antibiotics for both animals and humans. In a 2019 study on global trends in AMR in low- and middle-income countries (LMICs), authors expressed concern that there is less publicly available epidemiological surveillance data from Uruguay, Paraguay, Argentina, and Brazil – since they are large meat exports – while Colombia is the only country with AMR in animals that is publicly available.[66]

The concern is that as bacteria become resistant to the drug, it survives and continues to grow. In the Americas, multidrug-resistant microorganisms are the leading cause of health care-associated infections. A manual launched by the PAHO/WHO and Florida International University (FIU) calls on countries in the Americas to set up programs to optimize the use of antibiotics as a way to prevent resistance.[67]

One recent study conducted in Paraguay's Asunción River found the same genes responsible for multidrug resistance in humans also existed in wastewater.[68] A study by Moreno-Switt, Rivera, Caipo et al. reported that in Latin America and the Caribbean, most of the AMR research on water was conducted in Brazil, Chile, Mexico followed by Argentina, Ecuador, Uruguay. Recently, researchers called for the urgency to study pathogens in Uruguay, Paraguay, Guatemala, Honduras, Nicaragua, and Panama because no published articles were identified in these countries.[69] In another global study, scientists took samples across 58 major city transportation systems in San Paulo, Rio de Janeiro, Bogotá, and Santiago where they found AMR genes were 10–20 times higher than that found in Baltimore, Paris, or Singapore. Authors used the study findings to call for improved management of antibiotics in Latin America.[70]

Throughout Latin America and the Caribbean there is a plea for better governance of AMR. By the end of 2019, 29 (83%) of the countries in the Americas reported developing national action plans to contain AMR, applying a multisectoral approach. In 2018, collaborative research provided practical guidelines for health authorities as well as recommendations for hospital managers and health workers on cost-effective interventions that tackle AMR. In Latin America, Bolivia, Brazil, Costa Rica, Paraguay, and Peru contributed data on the sale of antimicrobials for human health to the "WHO Report on Surveillance of Antibiotic Consumption, 2016–2018."[71]

AMR is an excellent example of the intersection of animals, humans, and the environment, known as a One Health approach.[72] The different stakeholders from medical professionals, veterinarians, farmers, pharmacists, environmentalists, politicians, and civil society all have a responsibility for the problem and need to be part of the solution. This requires greater local to global collaboration, surveillance, improved diplomatic efforts with timely sharing of information for a security response to prevent, detect, and respond. Applying a Planetary Health analysis will provide a more holistic approach to such health security challenges. It begins with accepting the interconnectedness of microbes to humans, animals, plants, and the ecosystem where air, water, and land are impacted. This co-exists with how human systems will respond through ethically optimized and effective communication from concept to action.

More Challenges for Health Security

Health security is inextricably linked to transparency and sharing timely information about an outbreak so that decisions for the earliest intervention can be determined. In the Americas, we know cooperation breaks down when countries are unwilling or unable to share health information due to poor health surveillance systems. For example, Cuba's secrecy extends beyond the microbial threats. In violation of the international law, Cuba (July 2013) shipped arms to North Korea hiding 240 tons of Soviet-era arms along with 200,000 sacks of sugar on the Chong Chon Gang, a North Korean Freighter.[73] Cuba initially claimed it was a donation of sugar to the North Korean people. Ironically, the embargoed arms were discovered on the ship as it entered the Panama Canal, probably around the same site where Cuba's scientific and diplomatic cooperation to control yellow fever and malaria made the construction of the canal possible. Such a veil of secrecy threatens health, safety, and security. In 2016 a health and medical condition known as "Havana Syndrome" involved U.S. and Canadian diplomats in Cuba suffering from brain injuries, hearing loss, and other complications while serving in Cuba. There are many questions and security concerns, while research suggests microwave energy as the cause of illness among diplomats and their families. This creates a new level of health and security threats that has also been identified in U.S. diplomats working in China. This takes us into an entirely different area of weaponry and is beyond the scope of this chapter. "[C]learly health and security challenges are intersecting with greater frequency and intensity,"[74] wrote Jonathan Ban. While Ban's intent was not directed at the frequency of microwaves, a new attitude about the consequences of health and security matters is necessary today with new technologies, weaponry, and laboratory advancements.

Biosecurity and Biosafety

One topic widely analyzed in the international security literature is bioterrorism and bioweapons, and their role throughout history. This is beyond the scope of this short book and brief chapter on health security, and it is by no means to minimize its importance.[75] What is important is recognizing a biological agent can be naturally occurring, unintentional, or deliberately released to cause harm. The Biological and Toxin Weapons Convention (BTWC) was signed on 1972, that same year Cuba claimed the United States violated this convention in dispersing a pathogen harming their sugar cane and tobacco crops. This remains unconfirmed. In 1981, Fidel Castro blamed the United States for the deadly dengue hemorrhagic fever outbreak that killed 158 people including children, calling it "Yankee Imperialism" orchestrated through a Central Intelligence Agency (CIA) plot. Nevertheless, Cuba continues to accuse the United States of using biological weapons to cause harm against Cuban people, animals, and plants.[76] With all that we know and do not know, accusations have circulated for decades that scientific research experiments by the Rockefeller Foundation and United States government were responsible for diseases spreading, unintentionally, or intentionally. This is why a brief discussion on both biosecurity and biosafety is instructive in the examination of newly emerging and re-emerging diseases.

The intentional spread of diseases through acts of bioterrorism and defensive laboratory vaccine research has generated wider attention since the post-9/11 anthrax deaths. Advancements in scientific biological research reveal how scientists have the potential to create more dangerous pathogens than existing in nature. Dual use research of concern (DURC) is research conducted for defensive purposes but has the potential of becoming an offensive biological weapon and presents a greater threat to the health of humans, animals, and the environment. Gain of Function (GoF) research will seek out ways to modify the biological component to create new properties, such that a microbe can become more transmissible and more virulent. The controversy on public health security research resulted when two prestigious influenza laboratories, one in the United States and the other in the Netherlands, independently conducted studies on the H5N1 avian flu. Both studies showed how the H5N1 bird flu could be transmitted to ferrets in a laboratory setting. Publishing such studies in scientific journals was deemed a security risk in 2011 and the National Science Advisory Board for Biosecurity after "review of the unpublished manuscripts describing NIH-funded research on the transmissibility of H5N1.... concluded that the H5N1 virus has greater potential than previously believed,"[77] and recommended removing items from their methods and results sections in their final manuscripts.[78] The principal researchers and other scientists prepared a joint release through *Science* and *Nature* journals where they "agreed on a voluntary pause of 60 days on any research involving highly pathogenic avian H5N1 viruses leading to the generation of viruses that are more transmissible in mammals."[79] In January 2012, ten top experts showed a variety of disagreements within the scientific community concerning infectious disease research and security threats.[80]

Bioweaponry has been important to health security studies from the ability to develop potentially lethal pathogens, to rogue scientists facilitating a terrorist act, or gaps in laboratory safety causing a lab-leak that can place researchers and communities at risk. Biosecurity refers to biological agents that are naturally occurring, released by human error, or caused by the deliberate misuse of dangerous pathogens to cause harm. While most of the attention focuses on biosecurity, it is biosafety that deserves equal attention. Biosafety includes laboratory policies, procedures, training, and adherence to safety such as air flow and personal protective equipment (PPE) where high-risk pathogens are studied in biosafety laboratory levels (BSL), BSL-3 and BSL-4, such as Ebola and pandemic flu strains.

The laboratory research controversy about bird flu H5N1 features research on highly infectious pathogens in modern day. This involves GoF related to giving the biological component a new property. This is controversial because when microbes are modified to create new proprieties, this could make such microbes more transmissible and more virulent and possibly resistant to existing vaccines or treatment. Such experiments cause concern with new disease outbreaks and where both biosafety and biosecurity must be considered: "Whether it occurs by a quirk of nature or at the hands of a terrorist, epidemiologists say a fast-moving airborne pathogen could kill more than 30 million people in less than a year," claimed Bill Gates at the Munich Security Council in 2017.

Deadly microbes have the potential to kill millions, generate extreme economic losses, and create political instability. These biological threats could be naturally occurring in the ecosystem, unintentionally leaked from a scientific laboratory, or intentionally created as a bioweapon. Understanding these different aspects of biosecurity and biosafety is important to preparing, mitigating, and responding global health threats. Increased development, urbanization, global travel, natural disasters and climate change, improved technology, access to information for good and bad intentions by scientists and nefarious actors reveal 21st-century health security challenges. Biosafety is even more important today since it is an essential component of the GHSA that seeks to build up laboratory capacities in countries for the early detection of diseases in the efforts to prevent, detect, and respond to an outbreak and prevent a pandemic.

Conclusion

Latin America and the Caribbean countries document chronic diseases as the top reasons for disability and deaths, with demographic, epidemiologic, and health evidence to justify more research dollars for noncommunicable diseases. Nevertheless, many nations in the region still face a double burden of diseases, where communicable diseases disproportionately impact poor and vulnerable populations. The de-prioritization of infectious disease research, based upon the epidemiologic evidence, exposes the gaps in broader-based thinking and why we need to do more. Health security is more likely achieved by embracing a Planetary Health approach that extends to humans, animals, plants, and microbes in the ecosystem with a careful consideration of how human systems respond politically, economically, technologically, and ethically.

Currently, the greatest global health security challenge since the 1918 influenza pandemic is upon us, and Latin America and the United States have the highest infections rates at the time of this writing (early February 2021). The coronavirus pandemic is exposing the unambiguous racial and ethnic disparities, environmental injustices, widening economic gaps, with fear-provoking political challenges for global health governance. The WHO/PAHO's updated IHR, detection of newly emerging and re-emerging diseases coupled with growing health disparities, sharing of viral strains, rise in drug resistance, and naturally, human error, or intentional spread of a pathogen all contribute to the securitization of communicable diseases. In the final chapter, I propose using the conceptual approach set forth in this book to examine the multidimensional and multifactorial analysis of COVID-19. This requires the wider scope of study that considers how global and, more specifically, regional pandemic outcomes are associated with development, globalization, disasters and climate crises, diplomacy, and security.

Notes

1 The Preamble of the Constitution of the World Health Organization was adopted at the International Health Conference on July 22, 1946. Official Records of the World Health Organization, no. 2, 100, and implemented on April 7, 1948.
2 Howard Markel, "Worldly Approaches to Global Health: 1851 to the Present, *Public Health* 128, no. 2 (2014): 124, doi:10.1016/j.puhe.2013.08.004.
3 Frank P. Grad, "The Preamble of the Constitution of The World Health Organization," *Bulletin of the World Health Organization* 80, no. 12 (2002): 981.
4 Jennifer Brown and Peter Chalk, *The Global Threat of New and Reemerging Infectious Diseases: Reconciling U.S. National Security and Public Health Policy* (Santa Monica, CA: Rand Corporation, 2003), 4.
5 Adapted from Anne-Emanuelle Birn, Yogan Pillay, and Timothy H. Holtz, *Textbook of International Health: Global Health in a Dynamic World* (3rd edition, Oxford: Oxford University Press, 2009), 11.
6 David Fidler, "Navigating the Global Health Terrain: Mapping Global Health Diplomacy," *Asian Journal of WTO and International Health Law and Policy* 6, no. 1 (2011): 1–43. We lack reliable data on the health and diplomatic effects of soft power initiatives; see Ilona Kickbusch, "Global Health Diplomacy: How Foreign Policy Can Influence Health," *The BMJ* 342 (2011): d3154.
7 Roland Paris, "Human Security: Paradigm Shift or Hot Air," *International Security* 26, no. 2 (2001): 88.
8 United Nations Development Programme, *Human Development Report, 1994* (New York: Oxford University Press, 1994), 23.
9 United Nations, *Declaration of Commitment on HIV/AIDS: UN Special Session on HIV/AIDS, 25–27 June 2001* (New York: United Nations, 2001).
10 The United Nations Development Programme's, *Human Development Report* Created the Opportunity for More Intersectoral and Interdisciplinary Ways to Analyze Security.
11 Human Security Centre, *Human Security Report 2005: War and Peace in the 21st Century* (New York: Oxford University Press, 2005), http://www.hsrgroup.org/human-security-reports/2005/overview.aspx.
12 Sabine Alkire, *A Conceptual Framework for Human Security* (Working Paper 2) (Oxford: Center for Research on Inequality, Human Security and Ethnicity (CRISE), February 16, 2002), doi:10.1.1.580.2805.
13 Sadako Ogata and Amartya Sen, *Human Security Now 2003* (Washington, DC: Commission on Human Security, 2003).
14 Sakiko Fukuda-Parr, "New Threats to Human Security in the Era of Globalization," *Journal of Human Development* 4, no. 2 (2003): 167–179.
15 Stephen Morse, The Rules for Viral Traffic," in *AIDS: The Making of a Chronic Disease*, eds. E. Fee and D. M. Fox (Berkeley, MD: University of California Press, 1992), 23–48.
16 William Aldis, "Health Security as Public Health Concept," *Health Policy and Planning* 23 (2008): 369–375.
17 Jennifer Brown and Peter Chalk, 7–12.
18 Jeremy Youde, "Enter the Fourth Horseman: Health Security and Internationals Relations Theory," *The Whitehead Journal of Diplomacy and International Relations* 6, no. 1 (2005): 193–208.
19 Colin McInnes and Kelley Lee, *Global Health and International Relations* (Cambridge: Polity Press, 2012).
20 For a thorough analysis on this topic where authors use a constructivist approach to global health, refer to Colin McInnes and Kelley Lee, *Global Health and International Relations*.
21 Ronald Labonté and Michelle Gagnon, "Framing Health and Foreign Policy: Lessons for Global Health Diplomacy," *Globalization and Health* 6 (2010): 14, and

Ronald Labonté, "Global Health in Public Policy: Finding the Right Frame?", *Critical Public Health* 18, no. 4 (2008): 467–482.

22 Jean-Paul Chretien, et al., "The Importance of Militaries from Developing Countries in Global Disease Surveillance," *The Bulletin of the World Health Organization* 85, no. 3 (2007): 174–180.

23 Special thanks to Col. Alfred (Al) Allen for submitting a Brief History of FEST to me on August 13, 2009, for a historical record, and for personal communication with me on July 21, 2010.

24 Ibid.

25 Ibid, and Alfred M. Allen, *Internal Medicine in Vietnam, 1965–72* (Washington, DC: Office of the Surgeon General and Center of Military History, United States Army, 1979).

26 Louis Theodore Dorogi, "The United States Army Special Forces – Walter Reed Army Institute of Research Field Epidemiology Survey Team (Airborne)," *Journal of Special Operations Medicine* 9, no. 2 (Spring 2009): 54–71.

27 Dr. Al Allen, personal communication.

28 Refer to Case Study 6.1.

29 Mycology is the branch of science that studies fungal infections.

30 World Health Organization, *The World Health Report 2007 – A Safer Future: Global Health Security in the 21st Century* (Geneva: WHO, 2007).

31 William H. McNeill, *Plagues and Peoples* (New York: Doubleday, 1976).

32 Jared Diamond, *Guns, Germs and Steel: The Fates of Human Societies* (New York: W.W. Norton & Company, 1997).

33 William H. McNeill.

34 Gerald Haug, et al., "Climate and the Collapse of Maya Civilization," *Science* 299, no. 5613 (2003): 1731–1735.

35 David Fidler, "Germs, Governance, and Global Public Health in the Wake of SARS," *The Journal of Clinical Investigation* 113 (2004): 799–804.

36 David Fidler, *International Law and Infectious Diseases* (Oxford: Oxford University Press, 1999), 19.

37 Andrew T. Price-Smith, *The Health of Nations: Infectious Disease, Environmental Change, and Their Effects* (Cambridge, MA: MIT Press, 2001).

38 Sherri L. Porcelain, "Health Security in the Americas: Newly Emerging and Re-emerging Diseases," in *Reconceptualizing Security in the Americas in the Twenty-First Century*, eds. Bruce Bagley, Jonathan D. Rosen, and Hanna S. Kassab (Lanham, MD: Lexington Books, 2015), 265–285, and Global Health Security, accessed March 5, 2014, http://www.ghsi.ca/english/index.asp.

39 Ibid Porcelain, and "Video: Tom Frieden on Fighting Global Health Security Threats," *Smart Global Health* (Blog), *Center for Strategic and International Studies*, https://www.csis.org/blogs/smart-global-health/video-tom-frieden-fighting-global-health-security-threats.

40 Global Health Security Agenda, *Report on Global Health Security Agenda (GHSA) Framework 2024*, https://ghsagenda.org/wp-content/uploads/2020/06/ghsa2024-framework.pdf, 2.

41 Ibid, 4. Note: As of this writing, only the chair declaration details were available, https://ghsagenda.org/wp-content/uploads/2020/11/FINAL-CHAIR-DECLARATION-2020.pdf).

42 The NTI focuses on the prevention of catastrophic events that impact populations and the environment which are associated with weapons of mass destruction such as nuclear, biological, radiological, and chemical weapons, and more recently with cyber weapons. The JHU Center for Health Security focuses on protecting populations and promoting community resiliency whether from disasters, epidemics, or pandemics. The EIU research division of the Economist Group, the publisher

of *The Economist*, conducts in-depth analyses for governments and businesses to forecast political and economic situations in countries and take into account such events.

43 Nuclear Threat Initiative, *Annual Report 2019*, 15.

44 See GHSI data, October 2019, accessed November 2019, https://www.ghsindex.org/.

45 Center for Health Security, *Global Health Security Index: Building Collective Action and Accountability* (Baltimore, MD: Center for Health Security, October 2019), and https://www.nti.org/learn/countries/.

46 Refer to both of Paul Farmer's books: *Infections and Inequalities: The Modern Plagues* (Berkeley: University of California Press, 1999) where he explores the determinants of HIV/AIDS in Haiti and Tuberculosis in Peru, and *Pathologies of Power: Health, Human Rights, and the War on the New Poor* (Berkeley: University of California Press, 2003) where he further develops an analysis on structural violence, HIV/AIDS, tuberculosis, and multidrug resistance.

47 Stefan Elbe, "AIDS, Security and Biopolitics," *International Relations* 19, no. 4 (2005): 403–419. Michel Foucault, "The Politics of Health in the Eighteenth Century, in James D Faubion, ed., Robert Hurley translator. *Essential Works of Michel Foucault 1954–1984*, Vol 3 (London: Penguin Books, 2002), 95.

48 United Nations Development Programme, *Development Report* (2000) and United Nations Development Programme, *HIV and Poverty Reduction Strategy* (August 2002).

49 Anabela García Abreu, Isabel Noguer, and Karen Cowgill, *HIV/AIDS in Latin America: The Challenges Ahead* (Washington, DC: World Bank/Inter Development Bank and Reconstruction, 2003).

50 Wendy Grenade, "An Unwelcome Guest – Unpacking the Tourism and HIV/AIDS Dilemma in the Caribbean: A Case Study of Grenada," in *New Perspectives in Caribbean Tourism*, eds. Marcella Daye, Donna Changers, and Sherma Roberts (New York: Routledge, 2008), 188–218.

51 Caroline Allen, Roger McLean, and Keith Nurse, "The Caribbean, HIV/AIDS and Security," in *Caribbean Security in the Age of Terror*, ed. Ivelaw Lloyd Griffith (Jamaica: Ian Randle Publishers, 2004), 219–250.

52 Kelly Lee and Anthony B. Zwi, "A Global Political Economy Approach to HIV/AIDS: Ideology, Interests and Implications," *New Political Economy* 1, no. 3 (1996): 355–373, as well as Denis Altman, "Globalization, Political Economy and HIV/AIDS," *Theory and Society* 28, no. 4 (1999): 559–584.

53 Octavio Gómez-Dantés, "The Dark Side of Cuba's Health System: Free Speech, Rights of Patients, and Labor Rights of Physicians," *Health Systems & Reform* 4, no. 3 (2018): 178.

54 Donald G. McNeil, Jr. "Cuba's Fortresses against a Viral Foe," *The New York Times*, May 7, 2012.

55 Sophal Ear, "Swine Flu: Mexico's Handling of A/H1N1 in Comparative Perspective," *Politics and the Life Sciences* 31, no. 1/2 (2012): 52–64.

56 White House Press Release, *Crawford Texas*, March 23, 2005, https://2001-2009.state.gov/p//wha/rls/prsrl/2005/69849.htm.

57 Joshua Partlow and William Booth, "Swine Flu Devastates Mexico's Tourism Industry," *Washington Post Foreign Service*, April 30, 2009, http://www.washingtonpost.com/wp-dyn/content/article/2009/04/29/AR2009042904650.html.

58 Sara Miller Llana, "Mexico City Returns to Normal as Swine Flu Restrictions Fade," *The Christian Science Monitor*, May 6, 2009, http://www.csmonitor.com/World/Americas/2009/0506/p90s01-woam.html.

59 Sophal Ear, "Swine Flu," 58.

60 Portions of this section have been adapted, with permission from Rowman & Littlefield Publishing (November 4, 2020) from Sherri L. Porcelain, "Health Security

in the Americas: Newly Emerging and Reemerging Diseases," in *Reconceptualizing Security in the Americas in the Twenty-First Century,* eds. Bruce Bagley, Jonathan D Rosen, and Hanna S Kassab (Lanham, MD: Lexington Books, 2015), 265–285.

61 Nathan D. Grubaugh et al., "Travel Surveillance and Genomics Uncover a Hidden Zika Outbreak during the Waning Epidemic," *Cell* 178 (2019): 1057–1071.e11, https://www.cell.com/cell/fulltext/S0092-8674(19)30783-4.

62 Personal Communication with David Taplin, who responded and conducted microbiologic studies in 1972.

63 David Taplin and Sherri L. Porcelain, "ValuJet Flight 592 Air Crash Microbial Risks in Recovery Team," *Health Safety Report,* May 21, 1996, and *FBI Law Enforcement Bulletin,* September 1997.

64 "Antimicrobial Resistance," Additional Information on Antimicrobial Resistance and Infection Prevention and Control. PAHO/WHO, 2018.

65 See the International Federation of Pharmaceutical Manufacturers & Associations (IFPMA).

66 Thomas P. Van Boeckel et al., "Global Trends in Antimicrobial Use in Food Animals," *Science* 365, no. 6459 (2019). doi:10.1126/science.aaw1944.

67 Pan American Health Organization and Florida International University, *Recommendations for Implementing Antimicrobial Stewardship Programs in Latin America and the Caribbean: Manual for Public Health Decision-Makers* (Washington, DC: PAHO, FIU, 2018).

68 Jarbas Barbosade Silva, Jr., Marcos Spinal, and Pilar Ramón-Pardo, "Antimicrobial Resistance: A Time for Action," *Rev Panam Salud Publica* 44 (2020), https://iris.paho.org/handle/10665.2/52731.

69 Researchers also remarked that countries have few publications on the topic, in Ecuador, El Salvador, Bolivia, Venezuela, and the Caribbean; see Andrea Moreno-Switt et al., "Antimicrobial Resistance in Water in Latin America and the Caribbean: Available Research Gaps," *Frontiers in Veterinary Science,* August 21, 2020, https://www.frontiersin.org/articles/10.3389/fvets.2020.00546/full.

70 David C. Danko et al., "Global Genetic Cartography of Urban Metagenomes and Anti-Microbial Resistance," *BioRxiv: The Preprint Server for Biology,* August 5, 2019, https://www.biorxiv.org/content/10.1101/724526v1.full.pdf, and Claudia Mazzeo, "Latin American Subways 'Highest Antimicrobial Resistance'," *SciDevNet,* September 9, 2019, https://www.scidev.net/global/news/latin-american-subways-highest-antimicrobial-resistance/.

71 Jarbas Barbosa Da Silva Jr., Marcos Espinal, and Pilar Ramón-Pardo, "Antimicrobial Resistance: Time for Action," *Rev Panam Salud Publica* 44 (2020): e131. doi:10.26633/RPSP.2020.131.

72 See the AMR literature on One Health.

73 Maria C. Werlau, "A Closer Look at Cuba and Its Recent History of Proliferation," Hearing Before the Committee on Foreign Affairs Subcommittee on the Western Hemisphere, U.S. House of Representatives, September 26, 2013.

74 Jonathan Ban, "Health as a Security Challenge," *Seton Hall Journal of Diplomacy and International Relations* 4, no. 2 (Summer/Fall 2003): 19–27.

75 See the excellent review by Seth Carus, *Occasional Paper 12: A Short History of Biological Warfare: From Pre-history to the Twenty-First Century,* Center for the Study of Weapons of Mass Destruction (Washington, DC: National Defense University, 2017).

76 Milton Leitenberg, "Distinguishing Offensive from Defensive Biological Weapons Research," *Critical Reviews in Microbiology* 29, no. 3 (2003): 223–257.

77 Cited in Sherri L. Porcelain, "Emerging and Re-Emerging Diseases." See National Institute of Health, "Press Statement on the NSABB Review of H5N2 Research," December 20, 2011.

78 For a thorough analysis of this case study, refer to Gigi Kwik Gronvall, *H5N1: A Case Study for Dual-Use Research* (Council of Foreign Relations Working Paper) (Baltimore: Johns Hopkins Center for Health Security, 2013).
79 Ron A.M. Fouchier et al., "Pause on Avian Flu Transmission Research," *Nature* 481, no. 443 (2012): 443.
80 Anonymous. "The Fight over Flu: A Proposal to Restrict the Planned Publication of Research on a Potentially Deadly Avian Influenza Virus is Causing a Furore. Ten Experts Suggest Ways to Proceed," *Nature* 481 (2012): 257–259.

Bibliography – Selected Books

Bashford, Alison, ed. *Medicine at the Border- Disease, Globalization and Security, 1850 to Present*. New York: Palgrave Macmillan, 2006.

Chen, Lincoln, Leaning, Jennifer, and Narasimhan, Vasant, eds. *Global Health Challenges for Human Security*. Cambridge: Harvard University Press, 2003.

Collin McInnes and Lee, Kelley. *Global Health & International Relations*. Cambridge: Polity Press, 2012.

Kahn, Laurie. H. *One Health- And the Politics of Antimicrobial Resistance*. Baltimore, MD: Johns Hopkins University, 2016.

McNeill, William. *Plagues and Peoples*, New York: Doubleday, 1976.

Myers, Samuel and Frumkin, Howard, eds. *Planetary Health: Protecting Nature to Protect Ourselves*. Washington, DC: Island Press, 2020.

Price-Smith, Andrew T. *Contagion and Chaos- Disease, Ecology, and Natural Security in the Era of Globalization*. Cambridge: Massachusetts Institute of Technology, 2009.

Zacher, Mark B. and Keefe, Tania J. *The Politics of Global Health Governance – United by Contagion*. New York: Palgrave Macmillan, 2008.

7

CONCLUSION – PUBLIC HEALTH AND BEYOND

Case Study of COVID-19

Earlier in this book, I recounted my first experience in Latin America as an idealistic volunteer in Colombia in the late 1970s. I learned more than I could have ever given back to the resilient young girls and women besieged by their determination to protect themselves and their children. Earning meagre wages as street sex workers, confronting the higher risk of diseases, targeted violence, and sometimes death, the indomitable spirit of these desperate women was my awakening that a single approach to reduce the risk of sexually transmitted diseases was more than simply the act of educating women or the male clients to use condoms. One would think they were ill informed about preventing pregnancy or disease. I quickly learned that a woman would make more money if she agreed not to use a condom. Try telling a humble mother whose child is sick and hungry that she should take less money and protect herself now and for the future, without providing alternatives. She will choose to save her child and answer her immediate needs. We could try and convince her to change this risky behavior. The reality is we need to listen more if we honestly want to respond to the structural and commercial determinants of population health. This is what happens when we fail to take the time to listen to the hushed voices explaining why an individual acts the way they do, and how populations will rally around similar ways of thinking. Don't blame the behaviors without recognizing these structural inequities. The art and science of listening may be very useful today as we observe behaviors concerning what a mother would do to feed and care for her children, even if it means placing her health and safety at risk. This is evident during the current coronavirus pandemic where women are disproportionately working in jobs that could increase their risk.

This concluding chapter, in part, is shaped by my most recent experience in Latin America. The WHO pronounced COVID-19 a public health emergency

DOI: 10.4324/9781003007401-8

of international concern (PHEIC) on January 30, 2020. It wasn't until I landed at the Miami International Airport on March 11, 2020 that the WHO officially declared this a pandemic, the first in history to be caused by a coronavirus. In early March 2020, I traveled to the Guna Yala indigenous territory Panama, a place that has become my unofficial second home. I knew I had a short window of time, recognizing the virus was edging closer. I traveled for personal reasons to participate in some last-minute planning for an event that was two years developing, with the hopes of pulling it off in 2020 fading as the news reported that SARS-CoV-2 virus had been identified in Panama City from a resident who traveled to Spain. I knew I would have to depart before the decision was made to shut down boat transport between the communities and the city. I spoke with the community leaders and decided to depart the next day. This was the right decision since the following day all boat transportation in and out of the islands ceased operations. After the 5 ½ hour boat and road crossings, I arrived in Panama City to find a much more chaotic place than just a few days prior. There was monitoring and screening already in place at the Panama City Tocumen International Airport, and yet surprisingly, the Miami International Airport had absolutely nothing in place. No questions, no screening, *nada*. I exited using a mobile passport application without delay and prepared to enter quarantine for two weeks due to my international travel. Then everything shut down. It was spring break at the university, which was first extended and then transitioned to a remote learning. Rather timely, I was teaching a Disasters, Terrorism, and Global Public Health course. I am writing this one year later as COVID-19 has become the test for public health, development, globalization, diplomacy, security, and modern-day disasters.

The SARS-CoV-2 virus presents an excellent case study to examine the arrival and spread of a pandemic within the broader context of national, regional, and world affairs. Needless to say, it would require an entire book to give this topic sufficient attention. For purposes of this conclusion, in brevity, I will show how the deadly COVID-19 disease exemplifies the complexity of public health and the underlying determinants, competing perspectives, stakeholders, and partnerships from local to regional levels. Understanding how this pandemic intersects in the region of the Americas with (i) economic growth and development fears leading to a great recession, with income inequalities exposing structural inequities and rising poverty; (ii) globalization and the spread of a highly infectious microbe, as well as trade agreements for goods and services and access to reliable information; (iii) disasters and displacement as climate refugees seek safer and securer living among growing insecurity; (iv) public health diplomacy to promote greater transborder cooperation such as access to available and accessible supplies, therapeutics, and a focus on vaccines through regional and global public-private partnerships; and (v) public health security by strengthening new forms of diplomacy and transborder partnerships to prevent, detect, and respond to deadly diseases. Framing COVID-19 as a national, regional, and global health security threat shows how leaders are reacting to safeguard their population, defend transborder threats, and protect their economies.

The criticism of public health actions today appears similar to what occurred in the 19th and 20th centuries. This includes protecting the economy to strengthen colonial or former colonial powers, shielding the West from the pestilence of the East, or maintaining status quo of the rich versus poor as a disappointing reminder how little we have progressed beyond the great advancements in knowledge and technology. I suggest the historic lessons about public health disasters are well documented and understood. It is the elements of cooperation and transparency that surrender to the pressures sanctioned by weak global public health governance. This exists within a global village where social, racial, ethnic, and environmental injustices threaten the livelihoods of people juxtaposed to the fears of economic losses, political expediency, and power relationships of governments. The entanglements of public health are not new. Recognizing the COVID-19 challenge, the WHO Director General, Tedros Adhanom Ghebreyesus recently said, "we need our collective knowledge, insights, and experience to answer the questions we don't have answers to, and to identify the questions we may not even realize we need to ask."[1] A year into the COVID-19 pandemic, there are more questions than answers.

Public Health

Hippocrates (460–377 BC) first wrote about the history of infectious disease epidemics. Greek mythology (circa 500 BC) recorded the curiosities of Apollo, the God of Healing. Apollo fathered a son, Aesculapius, who became the God of Medicine, and fathered two daughters, Hygeia and Panacea. "It is said that he preferred Panacea. That he should have preferred the 'universal remedy' to the personification of health may have ensured his reputation among doctors but meant that Hygeia had to fight harder for recognition."[2] This fight is no different today.

The term epidemic gained prominence with Thomas Lodge's, *A Treatise of the Plague* (1603), and Gideon Harvey (1666) who used the term pandemic in his, *Anatomy of Consumption* (*Morbus Anglicus*) that refers to what is known as tuberculosis. The historical narrative of great plagues, such as the Black Death in London (1665), documents the earlier movement of diseases within and across states and regions of the world. The terms of epidemic and pandemic were used without suitable clarification until Frank Clemow (1894) presented the wide-spreading influenza pandemic[3] where the Greek word for pandemic, *pan* meaning all and *demos* upon people. From cholera to plague the first case of bubonic plague in the Americas was identified in Santos, Brazil in October 1899.[4] In earlier chapters we recognized the great successes in controlling the spread of infectious diseases along with the epidemiologic and health transitions taking place in Latin America and the Caribbean while also acknowledging that infectious diseases continue to disproportionately impact the poor and marginalized populations with further concerns about the newly and re-emergence of infectious diseases in modern times.

One of the greatest 20th-century global public health transitions may have occurred when the U.S. Surgeon General, Dr. William Stewart (1966–1969) claimed, "It is time to close the book on infectious diseases and declare the war against pestilence won."[5] Spellberg and his colleagues reported that even though this statement has been widely quoted, there are different dates, and no primary source for this great misstep in history.[6] This critical juncture in history influenced public health research and policy agendas as epidemiologic evidence revealed increasing rates of chronic diseases in rich and poor countries. It transferred the focus from communicable to noncommunicable diseases, while advocating for a new public health movement away from deadly bugs toward contemporary issues of lifestyles, tobacco, and unhealthy fats associated with chronic diseases.

The spread of newly emerging and re-emerging infectious diseases from animals to humans, known as zoonotic diseases, has become more important to global public health and the broader interactions of humans, animals, plants, microbes, and the environment. The One Health approach engages veterinary and human medicine, and environmental disciplines to work together to respond to the zoonotic diseases, causing more than 70–80% of newly identified infectious diseases in humans. A call for a more robust Planetary Health approach suggests there is a responsibility with ethical and moral reasoning to operationalize the urgency of human systems and respond to the changing ecosystem demands.[7] This includes ethical and factual communication regarding public health issues that may be lost in technical jargon, data, and arrogance. This happens too often when assuming people will react to the experts, just because it is said or scientifically validated. The coronavirus pandemic is the wakeup call long overdue in the study and practice of population health, safety, and security.

The first case of COVID-19 in Latin America was identified in São Paulo, Brazil on February 26, 2020 and continued to spread throughout the region. In November 2020, Latin America reported 33% of all COVID-19 cases and death, while the region only accounts for 8% of world's population.[8] By the end of 2020, Latin America and the Caribbean reported more than 15 million confirmed cases and more than 500,000 deaths. With each country responding differently it is difficult to provide a coherent regional approach to the pandemic. What we do know is that the COVID-19 pandemic struck Latin America and the Caribbean at a time of surging poverty, unmistakable inequality, and a defraying of social and political cohesion. Many countries in the region have weak and fragmented health systems, which do not guarantee the universal access to health care needed to address the COVID-19 crisis.[9]

The underlying determinants discussed throughout this book are observed across Latin America and the Caribbean. One clear example was discussed by Patty J. Davis, Dean of the School of Public Health at Cayetano Heredia University in Lima, who addressed the country's political instability since 2017, resulting in nine different ministers of health and four presidents in just a few years. She would know since she served as one of the ministers of health during such political uncertainty. She puts forth how a fragmented and under-funded health care system, weakened by political instability and lack of funding only exacerbated delays and logistical hurdles to meet populations' needs.[10]

Good public health practices respect testing, surveillance, tracing of positive cases and contacts, while promoting social distancing, hand washing, and face masks. This is not easy to implement in many countries where technologies are not widely available, and further challenged by limitations with physical spacing and lack of access to water and hygienic supplies. The luxury of physical distancing in crowded spaces with limited rooms, or consistent water, or resources for cleaning supplies requires more thought in the appropriate messaging where the underlying factors of housing, water, sanitation, and economic limitations exist. These are real hardships faced by many poor and indigenous populations across remote to peri-urban and urban communities. For example, an indigenous family I've known since the 1980s moved from their remote village to the outskirts of Panama City decades ago when my friend was diagnosed with cancer. Today she is cancer free; however, throughout the years she and her family confronted continual social and economic struggles raising and educating her children in an expensive city for low-wage earners often discriminated, while working in restaurants, hotels, or itinerant jobs. In a telephone conversation in early January 2021, I learned that her family has been without employment for ten months and was forced to depend upon the government food subsidies. She, along with members of her family, fears the virus, knowing many people who have died, and yet, they also fear the vaccine. At the time of this writing (February 2021), they do not have access to vaccines and when they do it is hopeful that a rigorous public health awareness campaign targeting vaccine skepticism will proceed the implementation of wide vaccination efforts. We have seen throughout history the great rewards of vaccines as a public good and ability to save lives. Vaccine hesitancy appears as a prevailing theme in responding to the pandemic. A culturally relevant campaign seems warranted well before the vaccines become available to the general population, rather than simply telling people what they *must* do.

One of the greatest contributions to public health, along with infrastructure investments in safe water, sanitation, housing, and nutrition, is vaccines. According to the PAHO (1995–2019) the Americas reported the highest vaccinations in the world, even though rates fell behind the regional targets. While global childhood vaccination rates are 85% for measles, mumps, and rubella (MMR), and diphtheria, tetanus, and pertussis (DTP), Latin America and the

Caribbean reports 94% rate of immunization for the first doses of MMR and 89% for DTP.[11] The COVID-19 urgency to develop, deliver, and get shots into arms demonstrates massive challenges while still maintaining the necessity of other preventive public health actions. For example, obesity and diabetes are comorbidities for COVID-19. The highest rates of overweight and obese populations are reported in the Americas. This includes the highest rates in the United States (68%), Mexico (65%), Canada, and the Bahamas (both documenting 64%).[12] Unmistakably, there are many population health issues placed on pause to allocate resources to fight the pandemic.

Development

The pandemic will continue to have wide-reaching economic impacts. According to the World Bank (2020), the global economy will confront the greatest recession since World War II, with an estimated per capita gross domestic product (GDP) decline in 90% of the countries.[13] The harsh impact of COVID-19 on development in Latin America and the Caribbean is expected to bring about 9.1% decline in GDP with the greatest declines in GDPs to occur in Venezuela (−26.0%); Belize (−14.0%); Peru (−13.0%); Antigua and Barbuda (−12.3); St. Lucia (−11.9%); St. Kitts and Nevis (−11.5%); Argentina, Bahamas, and Grenada projections are all the same at (−10.5%).[14] This captures the already vulnerable economies in the Caribbean with small states confronting disasters and climate crisis.

With increasing debt across the region, countries are spending to meet basic needs during the pandemic, further stressing their national budgets. Countries are creating innovative practices to meet the personal and financial demands such as placing a pause on tariffs related to medical product. Colombia, for example, eliminated value-added tax (VAT) on all products useful to managing COVID-19.

The Economic Commission on Latin America and the Caribbean (ECLAC) estimates 231 million people in the region are living in poverty, which is approximately 37% of the total population where extreme poverty will increase from 67.7 million to 96.2 million, reaching 15.5% of the total population in dire poverty.[15] The ECLAC further identifies the greatest increases in poverty are occurring in Argentina, Brazil, Ecuador, Mexico, and Peru with extreme poverty following in Brazil, Colombia, Ecuador, El Salvador, Mexico, and Nicaragua. Executive Secretary of the ECLAC, Alicia Bárcena, suggests the pandemic could reverse a decade of progress.[16] As discussed in Chapter 2, Latin America and the Caribbean remains one of the most unequal regions of the world with evidence of increasing inequality and rising rates of poverty associated with this pandemic.

And the economic outlook is not encouraging. Declining trade, weaker economic productivity, lower employment, and reduction in remittance from abroad will all contribute to further risks of increasing poverty. Regional unemployment in 2020 is estimated to be more than 13% with an estimated 44 million out of work. This is double to the previous year. Unstable markets and informal labor will make families more vulnerable. This is expected to be more damaging to Central American countries like El Salvador and Honduras where remittances account for 20% of the GDP, and in Haiti 33% of their GDP.[17]

As seen in earlier chapters, social protection remains essential for population health, especially in the provision of safety nets for the most vulnerable. Mexico's long history of social protection programs have a wide-reaching loan benefit program in response to the risk of high rates of joblessness across the informal employment sector. Dominican Republic's labor assistance program is providing job security during COVID-19 through the *Fondo de Asistencia Solidaria al Empleado* (FASE – Employee Solidarity Assistance Fund) as are other countries in the region. Supporting such development policies while protecting human rights will be a necessary approach to sustainable development in the region.

Education is one of the key elements of social development, and it is especially noteworthy in times of COVID-19. The pandemic is expected to have the greatest impact on children and adolescents, with an increased risk to the health, education, and safety of the most vulnerable population, such as the poor and Indigenous peoples. According to the UNICEF, eight months into the pandemic, 97% of the children in Latin America and the Caribbean have not returned to classrooms with four times more days of school lost than in any other region in the world. Distance learning highlights the disparities in learning where 75% of private schools have access to remote learning while rates are less than 50% in public school systems. During the 38th session of the ECLAC, held in Costa Rica from October 26 to 28, 2020, foreign ministers and other leaders throughout Latin America and the Caribbean convened to respond to the pandemic and sustainable development:

> While recognizing that substantial digital divides and data inequalities exist within and among countries and regions, and between developed and all developing countries, and that many developing countries lack affordable access to information and communications technologies, calls upon States and all relevant stakeholders to reaffirm their commitment to bridging digital and knowledge divides to promote research and capacity-building initiatives, as well as to enhance cooperation on and access to science, innovation, technologies, technical assistance and knowledge-sharing, including through improved coordination among existing mechanisms, especially with developing countries, in a collaborative, coordinated and transparent manner to help bridge those digital divides.[18]

Another concern is the infrastructure of schools where one in six of the schools does not have access to water. The availability and accessibility of safe water, sanitation, and environmental hygienic practices will be necessary for return to school during the pandemic.[19]

The diversity of populations and hierarchy of needs in this pandemic are a conspicuous reminder of how population welfare is closely interconnected to the social, cultural, economic, political, environmental, ecological, and technological determinants from urban to rural and rich to poor populations. Discussions remain focused on protecting the disadvantaged populations and seeking best practices to reduce their risks. As stated, many public health triumphs have been associated with vaccinations, as long as such vaccines are a global public good. This means that vaccines are nonrivalrous and nonexclusionary; yet the reality of equal access for all today is not a reality across rich and poor countries, equally. This may be different a few months from now. But sadly, we cannot say at this point in time that COVID-19 vaccines are performing as a public health good.

Burdened by mismanagement and corruption, with entrenched inequalities from income to education to employment to access to health protection, all present the wicked public health issues due to COVID-19. On October 28, 2020, the UN Economic Commission for Latin America and the Caribbean met to further support the COVID-19 response, agreeing to provide better social protections to tackle the inequalities across the region, even among those countries with increasing economic growth. Enforcing public health actions through laws, policies, and procedures, exposes the ethical challenges that communities may face when individuals or groups fail to adhere to such mandates. Bioethicist, Ken Goodman remarks, it is "The ethical foundations of public health standards, laws and mandates – all intended to protect society – make clear that individuals have neither the right nor the liberty to sicken their compatriots."[20] Furthermore, it recognizes that a human rights-based approach provides the context to question the moral and ethical decisions behind some dubious public health practices in countries. For example, Venezuela, El Salvador, and Paraguay forced thousands of people into mandatory quarantine in state-owned facilities with poor unsanitary conditions, lack of safe water, food, and health care. According to the Amnesty International, some of the restrictions were used as punishment for political opponents.[21] This is why science-based decisions in public health – and not the rationalization to support political agendas – are necessary to protect and secure society.

Globalization

The economies of Latin America and the Caribbean are suffering from reduced global travel, trade in goods and services, and a greater impact on the tourism industry. According to the UN World Tourism Organization data, international tourism declined during the first quarter of 2020 by 35% in South and Central America and 39% in the Caribbean when compared to the prior year.

Food importation is particularly an area of concern across the Caribbean where many countries such as the Bahamas, Antigua and Barbuda import more than half of their food. Regional exports showed declines of more than 25% during the same period. This is all further complicated by lock downs to targeted shut-downs, with mandatory isolations and closures of borders. Pauses in trade and interruption of the supply chain occurred throughout the region through 2020, creating economic disruptions within countries and personal economic devastation across populations.[22] This is not only about protecting population health at the expense of rising inequalities and economic devastation or neglecting the issues of environmental injustice and political turmoil. It is also about the interlocking problems that extend well beyond the health issue and ultimately impact the welfare and security of peoples.

The ECLAC political declaration further calls to:

> Emphasize that the COVID-19 pandemic has disrupted the normal func-tioning of open markets, global supply chain connectivity and the flow of essential goods, and that these disruptions hinder the fight against poverty, hunger and inequalities…reaffirms that emergency measures must be tar-geted, proportionate, transparent and temporary, that they must not create unnecessary barriers to trade or disruption to global supply chains, and that they must be consistent with World Trade Organization rules, and calls upon Member States to reaffirm the critical importance of connected global supply chains in ensuring the unimpeded flow of vital medical and food supplies and other essential goods and services across borders.[23]

Early in the pandemic, with escalating fears, xenophobia, and minimal data to make evidence-based decisions, a haphazard approach positioned some coun-tries against one another. The race to close borders, focus on a muscular vaccine strategy, and condemnation of the Chinese government spread throughout the globe. This was followed by the demand for better monitoring of trade in wildlife goods, and the closer surveillance of wet markets, raising worldwide concerns about the increasing spillover of infectious diseases from animals to humans. A wet market in Wuhan, China was first identified as the origin of the pandemic, where it was assumed an infected pangolin, a scaly anteater like animal, contracted the virus from an infected bat. Pangolins are one of the most highly traded animal delicacies eaten in China and Vietnam with black market prices as high as $1,000 a pound. However, this hypothesis has been refuted by many scientists. As of this writing the origin of SARS-CoV-2 virus is still in question. The assumption that it is a naturally occurring spillover event from animal to human transmission, or a potential Wuhan lab-leak, to numerous conspiracy theories with no scientific evidence. All this is occur-ring because there is a lack of transparency about the origin of SARS-CoV-2, with roadblocks to the access of reliable information within the complexities and weaknesses of global public health governance. This should be no surprise since 103 years later there is no agreement on where the deadly 1918 influenza pandemic began, even though it is sometimes referred to as the Spanish Flu. According to John Barry's, *The Great Influenza: The Epic Story of the Deadliest Plague in History* (2004), historians have presented competing hypotheses from British scientists saying it originated in a British Army Base in France in 1916, others suggesting Asia, and still others see it as occurring among Chinese or Vietnams laborers entering United States or France. Spain played a neutral role in WWI, and published accounts about the epidemic while other countries were censored from doing so. Consequently, labeling the 1918 influenza pandemic as the Spanish Flu is not accurate, since it more likely represents Spain's transparency though countries failed to do the same. Controlling the spread of diseases within and across the borders remains a challenge with quicker and further movement of people and goods as well as changes in behavior at time of travel, tourism, and trade. This gives rise to both communicable and non-communicable diseases, as discussed in Chapter 3, "Globalization and Public Health".

Trade agreements and public-private partnerships for supplies, medicines, and vaccines are ever more apparent during a pandemic. To exemplify, the demand for vaccines with this new vaccine platforms, known as messenger RNA (mRNA) platforms, requires it to be kept at $-25°$ to $-15°C$ (-13 F to -5 F) in cold chains. This presents great challenges for trade, transport, and timely reach in tropical and semi-tropical countries and more remote communities, unless greater investments in vaccine developments are made within a country. Thus, making such vaccine platforms is an unlikely choice for many areas in Latin America and the Caribbean. New technology provides both the opportunities and challenges for trade, albeit not always equally. To avoid redundancy, I direct the reader to Chapter 3 for the wider discussion on trade and public health, key stakeholders, and such issues relevant to the current pandemic.

Disasters and Climate Crisis

Confirming the origin of an epidemic that may become a pandemic cannot always be determined. Diverging hypotheses about where a public health disaster started have been documented throughout history. I mentioned the 1918 influenza above; however, the origin of the 1880s influenza, sometimes referred to as the Chinese influenza, is still disputed. An assumption "that extensive floods occurring in China might have started an atmospheric wave of disease-producing materials, which spread around the globe as the dust from the Java earthquake is supported to have spread, has not met with the general acceptance."[24] Throughout history the association of disasters and the spread of infectious diseases remain important when public health practices are not put into place. Using a disaster management approach for the current public health pandemic is both necessary and undervalued. Chapter 4 on disasters and climate crisis applied examples to show how an emergency event must encompass more than the medical and public health sectors to bring actions and policies to meet the demands for population health, safety, and security. This rests upon the planning, mitigation, preparedness, and resiliency that are central to public health prevention strategies. Without understanding the broader political, economic, social, environmental, and technological circumstances it is difficult to know how such events may take its toll on the welfare of populations.

COVID-19 is the greatest public health disaster in more than a century. This is occurring in Latin America and the Caribbean; while the climate, environmental, and economic crisis exists, political conflicts and increased inequalities continue. The pandemic struck as an ongoing migration crisis was underway with thousands fleeing Venezuela arriving across border in Colombia. This is taking place while Central America caravans are moving North, fleeing violence, poverty, and food insecurity. Faced with displacements from natural disasters and a climate crisis, mitigating further movements will require increased attention to policies to strengthen the resiliency of vulnerable populations. The political declaration in Latin America and the Caribbean called for increased finances to support mitigation, and adaptions for climate-resiliency.[25] In order to fund this, the foreign ministers and leaders in Latin America and the Caribbean countries met virtually to discuss new finance mechanisms such as Debt Relief/Swap for Climate Adaption for the Caribbean[26] as well as encouraging member states to adopt a climate and environmental approach to the pandemic recovery strategies that will help meet the Sustainable Development Goals set forth for 2030.[27]

Natural disasters, climate, conflicts, and pandemics often require innovative strategies for communities to meet the needs of educating children and their social development. School disruption in Central America has been further complicated by two devastating hurricanes, Hurricane Eta (early November 2020) followed shortly after by Hurricane Iota (mid-November 2020) wreaking havoc in communities in Belize, Costa Rica, El Salvador, Guatemala, Honduras, and Panama. This left many thousands of families displaced, and more than 1,200 schools damaged or destroyed in Honduras, Guatemala, and Nicaragua. Sadly, these are the same communities with the most extreme levels of poverty and violence throughout the region as this pandemic stalls development.[28]

To meet the educational needs of the most vulnerable populations during this pandemic, strategies could be adapted like used during other humanitarian crises. In a mid-1990s collaboration between the UNICEF and the United Nations Educational, Scientific and Cultural Organization (UNESCO), a School-in-a-Box Kit based upon the international standards of competency learning was created. The purpose of this kit was to maintain the continuity of education for children who were displaced from their homes or placed in refugee settlements. By the start of the 21st century, I learned more about how the School-in-a-Box Kit collaboration could be used in post-emergency events around the globe while serving as the Board Chair for U.S. Fund for UNICEF in South Florida. In 2002, we launched a campaign to create awareness and raise funds for such educational kits for children in Afghanistan where one in every two children is malnourished, only 6% has access to safe water, 10% enjoys adequate sanitation, and millions under the age of 15 are not able to read or write. Each educational kit was placed into a metal storage box weighing approximately 115 pounds and costing $300; this method was culturally and linguistically adapted to give access to essential educational tools for teachers and 80 students. Newer versions have added School-in-a-Carton as refill kits as needed. While it gained momentum in Afghanistan in 2002, the kit was also used among displaced populations in Colombia where classes could be held outdoors, under trees, or in open spaces. This seems appropriate for areas with limited access to technology, population displacement due to conflict or climate crisis, while efforts for more modern connectivity with financial support to keep students engaged remain a challenge. During the COVID-19 crisis, UNICEF in collaboration with countries throughout the region has found ways to continue educating children through radio distance learning programs, and other locally adapted strategies. UNICEF's regional report (2020) shares numerous interventions throughout the region. To exemplify in Peru's Ucayali region of the Amazon, loudspeakers reach students with limited internet connectivity. In Nicaragua, resources to purchase computers, cell phones, and data cards have helped children with disabilities through WhatsApp, video, and phone access for virtual therapies. In rural, indigenous, and other areas affected by conflict in Colombia, radio, television, and print materials assist in local educational needs.[29]

The other focus is getting people immunized. The shot in the arm approach identifies the weaknesses within a global response system. The first country in Central America to receive vaccines was Costa Rica followed by Panama; however, by mid-January 2021, the availability and accessibility through trade agreements show Argentina as having the highest rates of vaccination followed by Costa Rica, Mexico, and Chile. The role of public-private partnerships to mitigate the devastation of the pandemic must include South to South, North to South, and multilateral cooperation, which are people-centered, with equity and respect for human rights and freedom.[30]

Health Diplomacy

While we have seen successful regional and global cooperation for public health throughout this book, gaps still remain, and more attention to health diplomacy is warranted. The *Alianza Latino Americana De Salud Global* (Latin American

Alliance for Global Health) has advanced greater cooperation with academics and governments, and "have left the PAHO at risk of insolvency through lack of solidarity."[31] We are reminded throughout history, how many middle-income countries in Latin America have been overlooked from the wider global public health agenda.[32] However, the COVID-19 crisis has prompted new cooperation and collaboration efforts from regional to global public-private partnerships for global public health priorities and actions. This can be seen through old and new forms of vaccine diplomacy.

The concept of vaccine diplomacy was discussed in Chapter 5. There is a great deal to unpack about equitable access to vaccines where diplomacy continues to hold an important role. For vaccination, the Global Alliance for Vaccine (Gavi), a public-private partnership, began in 2000 with funding from the Bill and Melinda Gates Foundation in collaboration with the WHO/PAHO and UNICEF. The purpose was to provide equal access to vaccines to children in the poorest countries in the world. The vaccine alliance was bolstered by another foundation that filled the gap; the Coalition for Epidemic Preparedness Innovations (CEPI), implemented in 2017, which was conceived with a more robust public-private partnership approach. The purpose of the CEPI is to provide financial support for independent vaccine research to fight against newly emerging infectious diseases. While the CEPI has invested in vaccine development for SARS-CoV-2, "the absence of a major coronavirus vaccine initiative highlights the ongoing underinvestment in global infectious disease preparedness."[33] The development of vaccines is further complicated by logistics, management, supply chains, costs, and equitable and sustainable distribution to reach all populations. There are many lessons to learn from the disaster management and response systems to engage the public-private partnership when competition and conflict may highlight unilateral over multilateral approaches, at least in the short term.

In response to the pandemic, the Access to COVID-19 Tools (ACT) Accelerator was created in April 2020. This was designed to facilitate equal access to diagnostics, treatments, and vaccines. The ACT began with the WHO, European Commission, and France coordinating with governments, scientists, industry, public health organizations, philanthropist, and civil society. Focusing on the issue of vaccines, COVID-19 Vaccine Global Access (COVAX) was founded with participation from more than 66% countries around the globe. In August 2020, 80 countries came together to support a COVAX facility, where in Latin America and the Caribbean, Argentina, Brazil, Chile, Colombia, Dominican Republic, and Mexico joined. The COVAX facility was conceived as a pooled procurement effort to ensure that there would be equitable access to vaccines using a shared framework. This strengthened the existence of Gavi, CEPI, and WHO/PAHO organization partnerships across rich and poor countries, with governments and the industry ensuring all nations would have access to COVID-19 vaccines. Countries joined either with their ability to self-finance or receive funding to acquire vaccines after safety and efficacy measures were established. The success was contingent upon funding and support with a combination of self-interest, humanitarianism, and equity to meet needs. As of early February 2021, COVAX has not hit its target to distribute vaccines to resource poor countries, fearing they will be left behind; some countries are now signing their own agreements with industries to purchase vaccines.

Just a few months into the pandemic, on April 20, 2020, the UN General Assembly officially adopted Mexico's President López Obrador's G20 Summit appeal of international cooperation to endorse equal access for all countries to therapeutics, equipment, and vaccines, once available. This was followed by Costa Rican President Carlos Alvarado's request to create a WHO Technology Access Pool as a source of information for greater access to research and development tools. In June 2020, the Brazilian Health Ministry signed an agreement with Oxford-AstraZeneca (UK) to produce vaccines within the country with partnership with the Fundacão Oswaldo Cruz. In August 2020 this was facilitated by the Jorge Lemann Foundation, a Brazilian billionaire's investment to build a factory to manufacture the vaccines. Mexican billionaire, Carlos Slim, agreed to fund the production of Oxford-AstraZeneca vaccines in collaboration with Argentina to be widely distributed through Latin American countries. In July 2020, the Chinese Foreign Ministry in a meeting with Argentina, Barbados, Chile, Colombia, Costa Rica, Cuba, Dominican Republic, Ecuador, Mexico, Panama, and Peru announced a $1 billion loan to assist the region with greater access to China's vaccines, Sinovac Biotech and Sinopharm.[34] On December 11, 2020, Mexico approved the emergency use of Pfizer- BioNTech vaccine as the first country in Latin America and the Caribbean to do so, followed a few days later by Panama, Ecuador, and Argentina. Pfizer-BioNTech vaccinations began on December 24 in Mexico, Chile, and Costa Rica. On December 30, Argentina became the first country in Latin America to give authorization for the use of Oxford-AstraZeneca vaccines and up to this writing there were four countries in Latin America approving Russia's Sputnik V vaccine.[35] The Russian vaccine, Sputnik V, received early use approvals in Argentina, Bolivia, Venezuela, and Paraguay while some countries questioned the efficacy of the vaccine with limited data transparency and without the authorization from the WHO. On February 2, 2021, in a *The Lancet* peer review journal article, the research on Russia's Sputnik V showed it was both safe and efficacious.[36]

Creative strategies in vaccine diplomacy are warranted to ensure that there is increased accessibility with equitable distribution that considers all populations. This must be accompanied by transparency, appropriate messaging, and cooperation between governments, industry, and peoples. History has shown this is not an easy path. Possibly, this pandemic could exacerbate existing distrust of governments, with corruption and political unrest creating wider human security challenges. Let's hope such post-pandemic crises will be mitigated.

Health Security

As I have shared throughout this book, governmental trust is one of the most fundamental elements to public health practices and without this confidence, population welfare is ephemeral. Distrust that one's government does not have the best interest of its citizens is problematic and likely to contribute to poor societal outcomes. Improving the expectations of a global health governance response to the pandemic could best be served by applying the Framework Convention on Global Health first introduced by global health legal scholar Lawrence Gostin. This proposes a reshaping of the global health priorities and governance, with a call for the improved coordination and stronger leadership under the WHO. This has developed into a more robust international legal framework as it relates to global health governance from local to regional to global levels.[37]

At the end of May 2020, the United States announced it planned to leave the WHO and direct global health funds elsewhere. The United States first argued that the WHO was ultimately responsible for not exposing China's deception and hiding information about the virus. Officially, on June 6, 2020, the United States withdrew from the WHO to become effective June 6, 2021. Many argued this would weaken health security while others reasoned this was a humanitarian as well as a national security misstep. Upon taking office in January 2021, President Biden reversed this decision and rejoined the WHO along with the U.S. commitment to the Paris climate accords.

One of the greatest misunderstandings is that the WHO, a multilateral organization under the auspices of the United Nations, has the power and funds to compel countries to take actions. The WHO is forced to depend upon official governmental data, when in fact other sources may provide more reliable information. The WHO was never conceived to have a supranational mandate. Changing policies to allow the WHO to use other information and data than official government-approved statistics would help the organization. We have seen how such economic, political, or reputational rationale to withhold timely information has been an ongoing struggle to encourage transparency while depending on governments to release truthful and timely data. As such, possibly, a reform of the powers would require a fundamental change to the WHO (1948) Charter.

The response to the COVID-19 pandemic is further complicated by the *infodemic*, which is an epidemic of misinformation that is spreading rapidly across the different communication platforms through social and traditional media, creating problems for successful community-based health actions.[38] There has been a great deal of talk about conspiracy theories and anti-vaxxer movements against all vaccination, while the current discussion on hesitancy and confidence with the newly developed vaccine platforms confronts new challenges. In 2011, the Strategic Advisory Group of Experts (SAGE) on Immunization created a working group for vaccine hesitancy, which "refers to delay in acceptance or refusal of vaccines despite availability of vaccine services," and is influenced by many factors. This gave rise to the 3C's Confidence, Complacency, and Convenience Model for Vaccine Hesitancy where trust and perceived risk need to also consider the determinants of physical accessibility and geographic accessibility, affordability, and willingness to pay out of pocket if warranted, and comprehension of vaccines associated with language or health literacy.[39]

This SAGE working group identified three overlapping components from the (1) contextual influences associated with historical, social, cultural, economic, political, or environmental factors, to (2) individual and group level where influences of personal perception of a vaccine or peer influences occur, and (3) vaccine or vaccination-specific issues related to the vaccine. One of the first comprehensive reviews of the Model of Determinants of Vaccine Hesitancy was conducted in Latin America to identify the key drivers.[40] Guzman-Holst et al. found that the contextual influences impacting confidence in the vaccine and refusals were associated with lower social and economic levels, education, advanced age, religious and cultural practices, and misinformation about vaccine or fear of adverse reactions.

Today, we cannot overlook how public health and security are also linked to the role of social media and spread of misinformation as well as disinformation which is intentionally spread to satisfy an economic benefit or socio-political justification. Clear and precise communication has always been essential for effective public health interventions. The global reach of social media provides quick dissemination of such valuable information, while it also allows for sharing non-science-based assumptions, rumors, or false information, unknowingly or deliberately. A better understanding about the different viewpoints, attitudes, fears, and the emotions of people must all be part of the debate. "But science alone is not going to change the minds of those with strong beliefs."[41]

The intersection of public health and security triggered a renewed threat with a "fake immunization" Hepatitis B program in Abbottabad, Pakistan in 2011. The purpose was to collect blood samples from Osama Bin Laden family members to identify DNA samples and his location. This generated great concerns about the future trust of immunization efforts, and also left Dr. Shakil Afridi, a Pakistani physician working with the United States, sentenced to 33 years in prison for his participation. Rumors spread, claiming unwelcomed Western influence in the region. This left many local Pakistani community health workers to repair the damage by engaging Aman leaders to ensure childhood vaccines could continue to protect the health and well-being of their children. The fear that vaccines were the West's approach to bring about harm or population control to the East was not new. In 2014, tainted vaccines were found in an already devastated Syria. Young children died immediately after receiving the measles vaccines, questioning if it was an unintentional or intentional act. The vaccines were later found to have been unintentionally mixed with a dangerous muscle relaxant, leaving many hesitant about giving vaccines to children. Vaccines save lives and with all our knowledge and science there is a rise in vaccine hesitancy, and the controversy continues.

The central issue of mistrust is not easily forgotten, in research and in inoculations in Latin America. The unethical and repugnant Guatemala syphilis disease study, led by the United States Public Health Service (1946–1948) scientist John Cutler, was exposed 64 years later by historian Susan M. Reverby who had previously written about the alarming U.S. Tuskegee syphilis studies. Her work revealed how experiments were conducted on prisoners, prostitutes, indigenous military men, and insane and institutionalized children in Guatemala.[42][43] On October 1, 2010 formal apologies to the people of Guatemala were presented by the Secretary of State Hillary Clinton along with a personal call from President Barak Obama to Guatemalan President Álvaro Colom. The egregious violations of bioethics and moral standards in research with the Tuskegee syphilis experiments on Black men in prison continue to provoke distrust in government research and practice, and "[T]he inoculation studies in Guatemala put the efforts in Tuskegee in context but can also increase fear of medical research"[44] that continues today. In the early 1990s Giovanni Berlinguer presented the bioethical issues with an increasing threat of new epidemics and "necessity for international solidarity in the field of health."[45] In a globalized world where diplomacy and cooperation are critical, research integrity and ethical practices are fundamental to achieving public health security for all.

Conclusion

Leaking pustules and the swollen agony of widespread smallpox infections captured the human face in communities, cities, and countries large and small. This was visible as were the cases of paralytic polio victims. Could this contribute to why a modern-day pandemic – without the ugly physical signs of disease in plain sight – allows some to deny or minimize its deadliness and devastation? As I proposed earlier in the book, seeing is believing, and it is much easier to get people to buy into actions if it is something they can see or touch rather than something that is microscopic and invisible to the naked eye.

COVID-19 is an existential threat, extending well beyond the capacity and responsibility of the medical and public health fields to respond. Today, it is often said that the current pandemic is as much a public health emergency as it is an economic and political crisis, and a social, racial, ethnic, and environmental injustice event. Based upon what we know throughout the history to modern times, it's not a surprise that such problems are interconnected (Figure 7.1).

The chapters in this book provide the reader with an opportunity to explore global public health challenges, considering some selected historical, empirical, anecdotal, and experiential methods with examples and case studies from Latin America and the Caribbean. Identifying the underlying determinants,

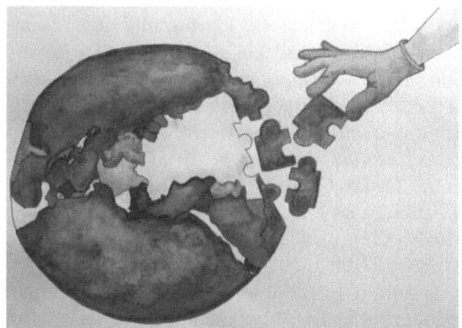

FIGURE 7.1 Public Health Puzzle for Latin America and the Caribbean. Design credits, Karina Rojas, March 2021.

competing perspectives of different actors at different levels of analysis, reinforces the emerging framework of this book. Furthermore, understanding how the socio-cultural, economic, political, environmental, ecological, ethical, and technological factors help to shape how we think and respond to the different public health issues. It is my hope that the reader will use a wider lens, embrace a kaleidoscopic approach, and seek further inquiry into regional to local public health matters be-yond the focus of the medical and health sectors. This includes a broader review of public health to development, globalization, disasters and climate crisis, diplomacy, and security with the eagerness to ask new questions and create your own puzzle.

Notes

1 World Health Organization and Global Research Collaboration for Infec-tious Disease Preparedness, *COVID-19 Public Health Emergency of International Concern (PHEIC): Global Research and Innovation Forum: Towards a Research Map* (Geneva: WHO, 2020), https://www.who.int/publications/m/item/covid-19-public-health-emergency-of-international-concern-(pheic)-global-research-and-innovation-forum.
2 Robert H. Bannerman, John Burton, and Chen Wen-Chick, eds., *Traditional Medi-cine and Health Care Coverage: A Reader for Health Administrators and Practitioners* (Ge-neva: WHO, 1983), 103.
3 Frank Clemow, "The Recent Pandemic of Influenza: Its Place of Origin and Mode of Spread," *The Lancet* 143, no. 3676 (1894): 329–331.
4 Walter Wyman, *The Bubonic Plague*, Public Health Service Bulletin #7 (Washington, DC: U.S. Government Printing Office, 1900), 6–7. Referenced in Loren George Lipson, "Plague in San Francisco in 1900: The United States Marine Hospital Ser-vice Commission to Study the Existence of Plague in San Francisco," *Annals of Internal Medicine* 77 (1972): 303–310, doi:10.7326/0003-4819-77-2-303.
5 Brad Spellberg, "Dr. William H. Steward: Mistaken or Maligned?" *Clinical Infec-tious Diseases* 47, no. 2 (2008): 294, doi:10.1086/589579.
6 Ibid.
7 See Samuel Meyers and Howard Frumkin, eds., *Planetary Health – Protecting Nature to Protect Ourselves* (Washington, DC: Island Press, 2020).

8 Pepe Zhang, *Moving Beyond Covid-19: Vaccines and Other Policy Considerations in Latin America* (Issue brief) (Washington, DC: Atlantic Council, 2020).

9 Relief Web, *Latin America & the Caribbean – COVID-19 Situation Report* (Relief Web, December 22, 2020), https://reliefweb.int/report/argentina/latin-america-and-caribbean-region-covid-19-situation-report-no-10-reporting-period.

10 Dr. Patty J. Davis, *Ensuring Everyone in the World Gets a COVID Vaccine* (Webinar Talk, Webinar, Duke Global Health Initiative, January 19, 2021), https://globalhealth.duke.edu/news/ensuring-everyone-world-gets-covid-vaccine.

11 Pan American Health Organization, *Core Indicators 2019: Health Trends in the Americas* (Washington, DC: PAHO, 2019), https://iris.paho.org/handle/10665.2/51542. See also Adriana Guzman-Holst et al., "Barriers to Vaccination in Latin America: A Systematic Literature Review," *Vaccine* 38 (2020): 470–481.

12 Pan American Health Organization, *Core Indicators 2019.*

13 Economic Commission for Latin America and the Caribbean, *Addressing the Growing Impact of COVID-19 with a View to Reactivation with Equality: New Projections*, Special report COVID-19 no. 5 (Santiago: ECLAC, 2020), https://repositorio.cepal.org/bitstream/handle/11362/45784/4/S2000470_en.pdf, and World Bank (July 2020).

14 Ibid, 9.

15 Economic Commission for Latin America and the Caribbean, *Addressing the Growing Impact.*

16 ECLAC was originally known by its Spanish acronym CEPAL. The commission was established in 1948 with specific focus on economic development of Latin America and then expanded to include the Caribbean in 1984 changing its name.

17 See the World Development Indicators (WDI)'s Online Database at http://datatopics.worldbank.org/world-development-indicators/, and Economic Commission for Latin America and the Caribbean, *Addressing the Growing Impact.*

18 Economic Commission for Latin America and the Caribbean, *Political Declaration on Sustainable, Inclusive and Resilient Recovery in Latin America and the Caribbean*, #32, https://periododesesiones.cepal.org/38/sites/pses38/files/political_declaration_of_latin_america_and_the_caribbean_-_final_23.10_ing.pdf.

19 UNICEF, "COVID-19: Over 97 Percent of Students Still Out of the Classrooms in Latin America and the Caribbean," *UNICEF.org*, November 9, 2020, https://www.unicef.org/lac/en/press-releases/covid-19-over-97-cent-of-students-still-out-of-the-classrooms-in-lac.

20 Kenneth Goodman, Director of the University of Miami Institute of Bioethics and Health Policy, WHO/PAHO Collaborating Center for Ethics and Global Health Policy, *Personal Communication*, January 19, 2021.

21 Amnesty International, *When Protection Becomes Repression: Mandatory Quarantines under COVID-19 in the Americas* (London, UK: Amnesty International, 2020), https://www.amnesty.org/download/Documents/AMR0129912020ENGLISH.PDF.

22 Economic Commission for Latin America and the Caribbean, *Addressing the Growing Impact.*

23 Economic Commission for Latin America and the Caribbean, *Political Declaration*, #18.

24 Frank Clemow, "The Recent Pandemic."

25 Economic Commission for Latin America and the Caribbean, *Political Declaration*, #21.

26 Ibid, #23.

27 Ibid, #29.

28 UNICEF, "COVID-19: Over 97 Percent."

29 UNICEF. "Education on Hold, A Generation of Children in Latin America and the Caribbean are missing out on schooling because of COID-19. November 2020) https://www.unicef.org/lac/en/reports/education-on-hold)

30 Economic Commission for Latin America and the Caribbean, *Political Declaration*, #14.
31 "Editorial: COVID-19 in Latin America: A Humanitarian Crisis," *The Lancet* 396, no. 10261 (2020): 1463.
32 Ibid.
33 Michael T. Osterholm and Mark Olshaker, "Chronicle of a Pandemic Foretold: "Learning From the COVID-19 Failure—Before the Next Outbreak Arrives," *Foreign Affairs* 99, no. 4 (May 21, 2020): 10–24.
34 I direct the reader to the timeline for a more thorough discussion on all countries in the region: https://www.as-coa.org/articles/timeline-latin-americas-race-covid-19-vaccine.
35 Ibid.
36 Ian Jones and Polly Roy, "Sputnik V COVID-19 Vaccine Candidate Appears Safe and Effective," *The Lancet* 397, no. 10275 (2021): 642–643. This is a review of Denis Y. Longonuv, et al.'s, "Safety and Efficacy of an rAd26 and rAd5 Vector-Based Heterologous Prime-Boost COVID-19 Vaccine: An Interim Analysis of a Randomized Controlled Phase 3 Trial in Russia," *The Lancet* 397, no. 10275 (2021): 671–681, doi:10.1016/S0140-6736(21)00234-8.
37 Lawrence O. Gostin, "A Framework Convention on Global Health: Health for All, Justice for All," *Journal of the American Medical Association* 307, no. 19 (2012): 2087–2092, doi:10.1001/jama.2012.4395.
38 John Zarocostas, "How to Fight an Infodemic," *The Lancet* 395, no. 10225 (2020): 675, https://www.thelancet.com/action/showPdf?pii=S0140-6736%2820%2930461-X, and Pan American Health Organization, *Understanding the Infodemic and Misinformation in the Fight against COVID-19* (Fact Sheet No. 5) (Washington, DC: PAHO, 2020), https://iris.paho.org/handle/10665.2/52052.
39 World Health Organization, "Report of the SAGE Working Group on Vaccine Hesitancy," https://www.who.int/immunization/sage/meetings/2014/october/1_Report_WORKING_GROUP_vaccine_hesitancy_final.pdf.
40 Adriana Guzman-Holst, et al.
41 Heidi J. Larson, *Stuck* (Oxford: Oxford University Press, 2020): 14
42 Marcos Cueto and Steven Palmer, *Medicine and Public Health in Latin America: A History*(Cambridge, UK: Cambridge University Press, 2015), 127.
43 Susan M Reverby, "'Normal Exposure' and Inoculation Syphilis: A PHS 'Tuskegee' Doctor in Guatemala, 1946–1948," *Journal of Policy History* 23, no. 1 (2011): 6–28.
44 Ibid, Reverby.
45 Giovanni Berlinguer, "The Interchange of Disease and Health between the Old and New World," *American Journal of Public Health* 82, no. 10 (1992): 1408.

Bibliography – Selected Books

Barry, John. *The Great Influenza: The Epic Story of the Deadliest Plague in History*. New York: Viking Penguin, 2004.
Basch, Paul F. *Vaccines & World Health- Science, Policy, and Practice*. New York: Oxford University Press, 1994.
Buss Marchiori, *Paulo* and *Tobar, Sebastián*. *Health Diplomacy and Global Health: Latin American Perspectives*. Rio de Janeiro: Editora Fiocruz, 2017.
Camus, Albert. *The Plague*. New York: Alfred A. Knopf, 1948.
Cardoso, Fernando Henrique and Faletto, Enzo. *Dependency and Development in Latin America*, trans. Marjory Mattingly Urquidi (Berkeley: University of California Press, 1979).

Cueto, Marcos and Palmer, Steven. *Medicine and Public Health in Latin America: A History.* Cambridge: Cambridge University Press, 2015.

de Salazar, Ligia Malagón, and Lugan Villar, Roberto Carlos, eds., *Globalization and Health Inequities in Latin America.* New York City: Springer International Publishing, 2019.

Diamond, Jared. *Guns, Germs and Steel: The Fates of Human Societies.* New York: W.W. Norton & Company, 1997

Fidler, David P. *SARS, Governance and the Globalization of Disease.* New York: Palgrave Macmillan, 2004.

Frank, Andre Gunder. *Capitalism and Underdevelopment in Latin America.* New York: New York University Press, 1967.

Garrett, Laurie, *The Coming Plague, Newly Emerging Diseases in a World out of Balance.* New York: Macmillan Publishers, 1994.

Gatti, Anna and Boggio, Andrea, eds. *Health and Development.* New York: Palgrave Macmillan, 2009.

Gilpin, Robert. *The Political Economy of International Relations.* Princeton, NJ: Princeton University Press, 1978.

Larson, Heidi J. Stuck: *How Vaccine Rumors Start-and Why They Don't Go Away.* New York: Oxford University Press, 2020.

Lee, Kelley. *Globalization and Health: An Introduction.* New York: Palgrave Macmillan, 2003.

McInnes, Colin and Kelly Lee. *Global Health & International Relations.* Cambridge: Polity Press, 2012.

McNeill, William H. *Plagues and People.* New York: Anchor Books, 1976.

Myers, Samuel and Frumkin, Howard. eds. *Planetary Health-Protecting Nature to Protecting Ourselves,* Washington, DC: Island Press, 2020.

Navarro, Vicente and Muntaner, Carles. *Political and Economic Determinants of Population Health and Well-being- Controversies and Development.* New York: Routledge, 2004.

Oldstone, Michael B. *Virus, Plagues, & History.* Cambridge: Oxford University Press, 1998.

Osterholm, Michael T. and Olshaker, Mark. *Deadly Enemies: Our War against Germs.* New York: Little Brown and Company, 2017.

Quammen, David. *Spillover: Animal Infection and the Next Human Pandemic.* New York: W.W. Norton & Company, 2012.

Vineis, Paolo. *Health without Borders- Epidemics in the Era of Globalization.* Cham: Springer International Publishing, 2017.

INDEX

Note: **Bold** page numbers refer to tables and page numbers followed by "n" denote endnotes.

United States: Chagas disease, spread
of 134; and Global Health Security
Agenda (GHSA) 168; and Global
Health Security Initiative 167; Global
Health Security Initiative (GHSI)
ranking of 169; as PAHO member state
24; score for biosafety 169; score for
biosecurity 169
United States Agency for International
Development Office of Foreign Disaster
Assistance 102–103
United States Public Health Service 202
University of Miami: Field Epidemiology
Survey Team (FEST) 102, 136, 158–161;
The Sue and Leonard Miller Center
for Contemporary Judaic Studies and
Middle East Peace Studies 146
UN World Tourism Organization 193
Uruguay: AMR research on water in
177; HDI score for 35; as member of
INCOSUR 135; as PAHO member
state **24**; smoking rates in 83
U.S. Agency for International
Development 102
U.S.–Cuba cooperation on Ebola 145
U.S.–Cuba relationship 140–144; cholera
denied 144; dengue and dengue
hemorrhagic fever to Zika virus
142–143; history re-emergence of
mosquito-borne diseases 141–142;
overview 140–141
U.S. Naval Medical Research Center
Detachment (NMRCD) 158

vaccine diplomacy 132–133, 198
Valdivia, Rivera 135
Venezuela: and COVID-19 vaccines 199;
as PAHO member state **24**; rise of
Christian democracy in 63
vibrio cholera bacteria 98
Vietnam: Field Epidemiology Survey Team
(FEST) 158–161; pangolins in 194
Vietnam War 158, 160
Virchow, Rudolf 18
The Voices of the Poor 38
Voices of the Poor from Many Lands 38
volunteerism: Haiti earthquake 114–115;
and health consequences 114–115
Von Meding, Jason 95

Wallerstein, Immanuel 37
Walls, Helen 84
Waltz, Kenneth 94

Washington Post 26
weather-related events 96
Weber, Max 37
Weisskoff, Richard 116
Welcome Foundation 137
western medicine *vs.* traditional medicine
25–30
WHA 62.15 129
WHA Resolution (WHA 61.21) 129
WHA Resolution 34.38 129
WhatsApp 197
WHO Codex Alimentarius Commission 79
WHO Technology Access Pool 199
WHO/UNICEF International Code of
Marketing of Breast-Milk Substitutes
74–75
WHO World Conference on Social
Determinants of Health in 2011 17
Witchdoctor's Apprentice (Maxwell) 26
women and economic development 52–57
World Bank (WB) 36, 38, 39, 41–43, 64,
167, 191
World Economic Forum Global Risks
Perception Survey 2017–2018 93–94
World Food Program (WFP) 89
World Health 65
World Health Assembly 74, 157
World Health Organization (WHO) 9,
22, 68, 70, 125, 153; Article 54 of the
Constitution of 125; Commission
on Social Determinants of Health
(CSDH) 39; Global Action Plan 176;
International Health Regulations
(IHR) 125, 167; Pandemic Influenza
Preparedness (PIP) Framework 133;
regional offices and PAHO members **23**
World Trade Organization (WTO) 64,
77, 167; International Centre for
Settlement of Investment Disputes 84;
Ministerial Conference in Doha, Qatar
129
World War I 24–25, 195
World War II 64, 166, 191

"Yankee Imperialism" 178
yellow fever (YF) 24–25, 125, 126–128;
background and history 126–127; today
127–128
Yellow Fever Commission 126

Zedillo, Ernesto 40
Zika virus 24, 34, 126, 142–143, 173–174
Zwi, Anthony B. 171